Also by Monica Grenfell

5 Days to a Flatter Stomach

• • • • • • • • • • • • •

MONICA GRENFELL

Fabulous
in a Fortnight

PAN BOOKS

First published 1995 by Montgomery Books

This revised edition published 1997 by Pan Books
an imprint of Macmillan Publishers Ltd
25 Eccleston Place, London SW1W 9NF
and Basingstoke

Associated companies throughout the world

ISBN 0 330 35368 3

9 8 7 6 5 4 3 2 1

A CIP catalogue record for this book is available from
the British Library.

Typeset by Set Systems, Saffron Walden, Essex
Printed and bound in Great Britain by
Mackays of Chatham plc, Chatham, Kent

● ● ● ● ● ● ● ● ● ● ● ● ● ●

To my late parents, and my beloved husband Michael

● ● ● ● ● ● ● ● ● ● ● ● ● ●

Acknowledgements

Grateful thanks to the following for their technical assistance:

Amanda Fredericks, ITEC, IHBC, OSH, Beauty Therapist
Toni and Guy Hairdressers, Oxford

Advice to the Reader

Before following any medical or dietary advice contained in this book, it is recommended that you consult your doctor if you suffer from any health problems or special conditions or are in any doubt as to its suitability.

Contents

Introduction

How's it possible to look Fabulous in a Fortnight? If you're two stone overweight, had a disastrous haircut last week, are tied to the house with three tiny children and a bucketful of dirty washing, or haven't enough money to buy anything more stunning than a new pair of tights, it'll take more like a Miracle in a Month to get you anywhere near fabulous. Right?

Wrong. Absolutely anybody can look fabulous. It doesn't take a healthy bank balance and it doesn't call for a string of beauticians or an extensive wardrobe. Most of us know someone who has all these advantages, yet still manages to look a mess. Every woman, from sixteen to sixty has what it takes to look good because that something comes from within. All you need to do is to recognize your good points, make the most of them, and not rely on clothes or jewellery to make a statement for you.

We've all been there. It doesn't matter if you're wearing the entire Paris Spring Collection and have boosted your income with a nice promotion. If you woke up feeling fat, you're having a Bad Face Day and your hair's gone wrong, the day will be a disaster.

On the other hand, we all know someone who can pull on a pair of jeans, tuck in an old shirt, run a hand through a mane of hair and look a million dollars. It's got nothing to do with clothes or being super-skinny. It's about style, and no amount of money can buy it.

Looking fabulous is all about *feeling* fabulous, and that means feeling confident. And it's hard to feel confident when you hide your neglected nails every day under another thick coat of nail varnish. Everyone papers over the cracks from time to time, but you can't live like that for ever. Why not? Because you're living for now, not in the future. Don't spend your life saying you'll do something about your weight *when* this busy period's over, or *when* the New Year starts. Don't keep telling yourself you'll sort your hair out as soon as your college course finishes, the children have started school or your divorce comes through. In the meantime you feel bad and your meter's running. Do something about it today.

You'll never get caught out

The Fabulous Woman never gets caught out. She looks fantastic in the legendary binliner. Even on a wet Saturday afternoon in the supermarket, taking the dog for a walk or putting out the rubbish, she looks great. My Fabulous Friend was once called out of bed in the middle of the night because her apartment building was on fire. Wearing an old T-shirt, no make-up and a slick of greasy night cream, she waited on the balcony for an hour while the emergency was quelled. Next morning one of the fire-fighters knocked on her door and asked her out. 'I think you're stunning,' he said.

High maintenance is out

We've all heard about High Maintenance Women. It's a good joke while it lasts, but some people actually live like that. Frankly, if it costs so much and takes so much time to get yourself into shape looking halfway decent, you're doing something wrong. And are the results really worth it? I've never been convinced, and in this book I'm setting out to prove that with a bit of organization and commitment, you can look Fabulous in Just a Fortnight without having to book into a health farm, spend hundreds of pounds or lash out on a whole new wardrobe.

• • • • • • • • • • • • • •

True beauty can't be taken off

Clothes count, of course they do. If you've worked hard on your figure, face and hair, the crowning glory is to put on something lovely and know you look terrific. Wearing something patently unflattering, over-the-top or unsuitable can also undo all your good work, so clothes *are* important. The general rule, though, is that if your look depends on something which can be removed, such as make-up or jewellery, you've gone wrong. If you're the sort of woman nobody recognizes without her face, you're going badly wrong. If you look sensational in your glad rags or best work clothes but a tip when you're weeding the garden, you're heading for disaster. We all have off-days. Looking a bit off is OK. Looking grubby and neglected isn't.

Being known for having a good dress sense is one thing, but you don't want to become an accessory to your clothes. If every aspect of your outfit can be described in detail but no one can remember the colour of your eyes, this book's for you.

This isn't a low-budget alternative for people who can't afford the luxury of salons. French women are taught from their earliest days to look after their own grooming and settle for nothing less than the best. I'm showing you the right way to take charge of yourself so you're always one jump ahead of yourself, and the competition.

These are the main elements of the Fabulous Woman:
1. She's slim.
2. She has good legs.
3. Her complexion is clear and healthy.
4. Her hair is glossy and healthy-looking.
5. She has cared-for hands and feet.
6. She has good posture.
7. Her body is smooth and scented.
8. She has a good bustline.
9. She has a bright and friendly smile.

• • • • • • • • • • • • • •

Over the next fortnight we're going to tackle all these elements on a day-by-day basis. Whatever you look and feel like right now, you're going to look better!

I have often been tackled on my belief that slim is better. Many bigger women say they're happy the way they are and I believe them. I say I'm happy with my height and couldn't care less about my narrow shoulders. What I really mean is that as I can't do anything about either of them I've stopped worrying and live with them, but given a straight choice with absolutely no effort involved, I'd bite your hand off for an extra two inches on my height.

Many of my clients come to me because they have a specific occasion in mind for which they want to look their best. It can be anything from a job interview or first day in a new job, the date of a lifetime with someone special, or the homecoming of a loved one. I even helped one young girl who was unexpectedly asked out by the boy of her dreams to watch him play cricket, and although she would be wearing casual clothes, she nonetheless wanted to grasp the opportunity and make the best of herself. She shed half a stone, her skin lost its spots, and it obviously worked because they're now engaged!

'I can't seem to meet the right man,' wailed one friend the other day, while another said, 'I can't meet any at all!' Is this you? Do you feel you spend most of your life worrying about your figure, your face, the length of your hair and every spare millimetre on your thighs, and STILL can't find a decent partner?

The truth is, women care far more about what other women think of them (which is why, for instance, many women actually compete to be thinner than one another). This form of competition is understandable in that results are seen to indicate achievement, but silly because it doesn't actually get you anywhere. When are we going to start listening to what men say they prefer women to look like? Men don't find thin women desirable, any more than they find fat women desirable. If you read men's views in the

What 'Fabulous' Means to Me section (page 11), you'll see that personality counts far more than body size, and if you look confident, radiant and happy, and have a healthy figure which is toned, cared about and carried well, men will be coming out of the brickwork.

My own field of expertise is diet, exercise and nutrition, and I have consulted some of the best beauty therapists and hairdressers in the business for their expert advice.

You WILL lose weight before the fortnight's out. You WILL tone up and feel fresher. You WILL have a clearer skin and a flatter stomach. Isn't that enough to be going on with?

You've got just two weeks!

I don't have time!

Women who've let themselves go always say that they haven't time. They are suspicious of people who manage to run a home, children and a full-time job and still look glamorous, and there's usually some bitchy comment about being able to afford it, having a mother-in-law to help, or a hen-pecked husband. It's only jealousy, of course. Everybody has twenty-four hours in a day, and compared to our mothers and grandmothers, who didn't have washing machines, microwaves or cars, we've got it made.

No woman who considers herself efficient should have to admit that she can't find time for herself. Even in the midst of your many duties and responsibilities you can keep your looks, your health and your youthfulness of face and figure. The trick is to organize yourself on labour-saving lines so you can easily find time to give yourself simple little beauty treatments and watch your diet.

The secret is not to be haphazard. I've designed the basic plan for you, but for the future you can find a way of incorporating my ideas into your own lifestyle. Designate a day for each task and discipline yourself to sticking with it.

• • • • • • • • • • • • • •

Say 'I'm going to exercise on Sunday, Tuesday and Wednesday, do my nails on a Friday evening and my feet on Monday morning. I'll pluck any stray eyebrows every morning and do my fake tan each Saturday' – or whatever timetable suits you. Do the same with meals. This plan tells you what to eat, but in future make a weekly menu. It takes all the stress out of it. Haphazard shopping leads to impulse buys of things you then have to eat up because they're in the way.

Doing it yourself

This book is about doing it all yourself. Top London salons charge around £255 for just one day of top-to-toe pampering and two weeks at a health farm will set you back hundreds, maybe thousands of pounds. Even if the expense means nothing to you, you can't just take a fortnight out of a crowded schedule without some planning. Maybe you live in the depths of the countryside and the nearest salon is miles away? Not everyone has a fully equipped gymnasium and leisure centre up the road, and if you're managing on a windswept smallholding with three dogs, a business to run and an elderly dependent relative, you won't thank me for suggesting you start the day with an aerobics class.

However, good reasons soon become excuses. It might be easy to organize yourself, but other people aren't so accommodating. I was a young mother once, frequently managing on my own when my husband was away, in a freezing cottage miles from the nearest town. In those circumstances it's easy to feel there's no reason to look good, but you must soldier on. Children grow up, circumstances improve. In my day exercise was a daily trot to the post office pushing a double pram, and two ten-minute sessions of stomach exercises, but being slim kept my spirits up. Try to incorporate daily exercise into your life, and it'll be like an insurance policy for the future.

• • • • • • • • • • • • • •

Have a good clear-out

The first part of this plan is the easiest. Start with a clean sheet tomorrow morning by throwing out the leftover chocolates, dregs of wine and that packet of sausages lurking at the back of the fridge. In fact, why not clear your fridge out completely? Then get a decent night's sleep followed by a trip to the shops for some proper nourishing food. After a spot of brisk exercising and a good scrub down, you'll be feeling a hundred times better, and it's only Day One! Then you really get down to it . . .

Tried and tested

In early 1996, I was asked by the BBC's *Good Morning with Anne and Nick* programme to help one of their viewers, Denise Peach, get herself ready for her degree ceremony. Denise worked full-time for the West Midlands Police Force and had three children and a home to run, and although she was an attractive woman with a wonderful personality, she understandably felt that with three years of studying behind her, she'd let herself go. When I met her, she was slightly overweight and neglected, with astonishing eating habits! She tended to skip breakfast, and her first food of the day was something chocolatey or gooey for elevenses. Needless to say, her main problem was bloating and lack of energy.

Denise followed the complete plan, with posture exercises, and had amazing results. She actually lost a total of twenty-three inches from her hips, thighs, stomach and bottom, and five and a half pounds in weight. Her inch loss was entirely due to her eating a good ceareal or toast breakfast, eating little and often and including plenty of water in her diet. Combined with the exercise plan, Denise rid herself of excess retained fluid and found all her clothes loose. Her beauty routine, too, had brightened her skin which was really blooming, and she looked radiant for her big day. I'm sure you will be thrilled with your results, too.

As I said before, the first day is easy, then you have to get down to the basics of looking fabulous. They are simple:

• • • • • • • • • • • • •

1.   EAT GOOD, PLAIN FOOD

'You are what you eat' is true. A diet which has too many additives, is a struggle for the body to process, and contains more calories than you need, will leave you spotty, bloated and fat.

2.   DRINK PLENTY OF WATER

There is nothing quite like plain water for improving your looks. You may not relish the idea, but on this plan you will be drinking six glasses of water a day *in addition to* your normal drinks, but the difference in your looks will be dramatic.

3.   IMPECCABLE GROOMING

However much make-up you apply, however many coats of nail varnish, however lavish your hairstyle, nothing can hide poor condition. A grimy, greasy or dry skin, rough cuticles, hideous heels, a dirty neck and lank hair can never be disguised. Keeping your grooming up together is a MUST if you want to look good.

4.   REGULAR EXERCISE

Exercise does more than just tone your muscles and help keep your weight down, important though these are. Exercise is a beauty aid. Good circulation results in clearer skin and healthier nails and hair. *Never* neglect your daily exercise, even if you find it hard to make time. Nobody was ever sorry that they took a nice brisk walk. People are only sorry that they didn't. Stretching exercise is vital for people who have to spend their day sitting down, or who for other reasons are inactive. Stretched limbs look leaner and a supple body is youthful. I accept that some women look fantastic despite the fact that they regularly drink half the Loire Valley, smoke twenty a day and only manage to walk to the car, but it never lasts. At my age, 'Have you seen the state of her?' is a phrase I hear weekly.

5.   DON'T BE TOO THIN!

Most women long to be thin. We've all heard the old saying 'You can't be too rich or too thin', but you can. Being too thin might not only leave you a cripple, but it can look ghastly.

A thin, pert little face is fine if you're twelve. It's not even too bad if you're twenty, but when you get to your thirties and forties it starts to look gaunt. From gaunt, it's a short step to looking stringy, and from there it's downhill all the way. It's not so bad if you've always been thin, but sudden weight loss in later years does your face no favours. Cheeks which used to be pleasantly plumped out become jowls, which means you lose your jawline, and the neck skin becomes loose. The effect on your bosom is obvious because breasts are mainly fat anyway. A push-up bra which is pushing up wrinkled skin is not a pretty sight.

You don't want to look young so much as youthful. Youthful means a bit of fat under your chest so you don't look like a toast rack in low-cut dresses. Youthful means a rounded face with a dewy complexion, and you can't get that on a fatless diet. Youthful means plenty of water in the diet to plump out those wrinkles as they appear. It seems almost too simple, but it's a fact. Skinniness – unless you were born to it and therefore it suits you – is not something to aspire to. On this plan we will concentrate on achieving a healthy, womanly, slim and toned appearance.

Over the next two weeks you're gradually going to feel more supple, groomed and trimmer, and that's the secret to feeling Fabulous in a Fortnight.

Find the time. *Make* the time! In just two weeks it's easy to turn yourself around if you have the will. Make your family understand that you wish to discipline yourself for a while, and try not to be too tense about it or it becomes an issue. Try not to tell the whole office or college that you're on a diet, or they'll either take the mickey or get fed up with you. It's a pressure on you if you fail to live up to your own expectations. Far better to have everyone whispering behind your back about how glowing and confident you look, and how on earth have you managed it!

More than just looks

One final thought. How often have you heard someone say that a girl was all right 'until she opened her mouth'? Or 'She ruined it all by the way she behaved at dinner'? Or some other scathing comment which suggests that beauty is more than skin-deep?

This book is not an attempt to change your ways and

personality totally, but we all have to acknowledge that sometimes it is our behaviour, or our speaking voice or general manner which can be offputting, and we are always the last to suspect. In case you think you might fall into this category, I have included a section on deportment and general carriage and another on behavioural mistakes most of us make at some time or another, usually when young. If your bubbly nature includes ripe language and extravagant behaviour, and you feel it has never held you back in any way, by all means ignore the advice and press on. However, if you are reading this book because you feel you somehow fall short in the popularity stakes, your relationships never work, and you never get asked to the right parties, you may discover this could be for some trifling reason you're not aware of. It's advisable to read this section (see pages 20–8) and see if something rings a bell. After all, you won't have lost anything. Impeccable manners, a lovely speaking voice and beautiful posture never let anyone down.

• • • • • • • • • • • • • •

What 'Fabulous' Means to Me

I've already said that the basic elements of a Fabulous Woman are good legs, figure, complexion, posture, hair and nails. Add to this a friendly smile and you have a base which nobody can take away.

But what do other people think looks fabulous? I asked a group of men for their opinions and here are the responses of a handful of them. See if you can find a common thread.

GARRY SAMMS, 19, is a student
'I think long legs are fabulous. Or if they aren't actually long, they should look like they are. I suppose that means slim. I don't care much if her legs aren't shapely, though it helps, I just can't stand legs like a footballer's, or big ankles. I also find a flat stomach sexy. Sorry!'

ANDREW, 44, is a newspaper and glamour photographer from Perth
'I don't want to sound pretentious, but it's what we used to call at college "aesthetic continuation". That means that a woman has many qualities which, put together, make her glamorous, but they don't all rely on each other. She can have bad hair, an off-day with her face or put on a few pounds, but the essence of her beauty doesn't suffer in any way. If someone is only gorgeous because of particularly stunning hair, or her figure, she's nowhere to go if they fail her, such as if she cuts her hair short or wears trousers.

'A woman should be able to make a lot of changes to herself and still look good, but I admit that it's rare to find someone with these qualities. My personal hate? Oh, believe it or not, I notice elbows and have a particular dislike for rough ones, or dry, "goosefleshy" skin on the back of arms and shoulders. In my job I see it all, and you'd be amazed how many models forget the hidden bits.'

MICHAEL, 38, is a safety manager at a car plant
'My mother always looked fabulous and she had no money for clothes. Her hair was always immaculate even though she never went to the hairdresser, and she sort of tap-tapped along in her high heels.

'She was a glamorous figure to me, despite her lack of cash. I can see her now, peeling potatoes by the sink, back ramrod-straight, smelling of perfume. If only women were like that nowadays.'

JEFF, 26, is a catering manager for a large haulage company
'A woman's fabulous to me if she smells nice, has a small bottom and a big smile.'

ALEXANDER JARVIS, 41, is a financial services consultant from London
'My girlfriend's fabulous. She goes to the gym a lot but she's not hung up about her figure, and I couldn't stand it if she was a fitness freak. She takes care of her body but still enjoys a good curry! She has a lovely glow about her when she's been training, and the skin on her thighs is so silky as a result.'

BOB WISEMAN, 32, is a painter and decorator from Cambridge
'My wife Janet is completely fabulous, and I always fancy her whatever she's wearing. She's always saying she should

• • • • • • • • • • • • • •

do something about her weight because she's about a stone too heavy, but that's her opinion.

'Her weight doesn't matter because she's got a fantastic personality. Even when things have been bad for us financially she's cheerful, and keeps us all from feeling miserable. I couldn't stand a woman who was miserable all the time. You can take so much, then it just gets to be hard work. Her smiling face is pure beauty to me, and she's very kind to other people too. I think that if it's obvious that everyone else thinks a lot of your wife, you do too. It's nice being married to a popular person.

'Janet has a good dress sense, and I see the same things year after year. She often says, "It's this old thing again": she can buy what she likes but still brings out the same dresses. I'm glad that she's not neurotic about it. She has a navy blue and white dress which looks sensational, and she must have been wearing it since the early 1980s, but if you look fantastic in something, why go and buy something else?'

BARRY JONES, 34, is a gamekeeper in Gloucestershire
'I love a natural look. Casual clothes, sporty and fit, that's fabulous for me.'

JAMES WALL, 19, is a trainee chef from Devon
'Clean hair, natural colour, no roots showing. When I see a girl with healthy, swinging hair, I think it's fabulous.'

JAMES LAVERS, 20, works in television
'Her smile. In my job I see a lot of models who are beautiful-looking, but they stand there looking bored or unhappy or just unsure of themselves. I can understand if you lack confidence because you've been caught without your make-up on or straight from the bath, but when they've done themselves up and still lack confidence it's not very attractive. I think a lovely smile is fabulous. And lovely clean hair.

• • • • • • • • • • • • • •

I'm not bothered about long or short, fair or dark, as long as it looks healthy.'

SIMON PARKES, 40, is a GP
'Smoking isn't fabulous, having fresh breath is. I also notice nice nails, though I'm not keen on talons or red nail varnish. Just nice and clean-looking will do fine.'

FREDDIE ALLSOP, 22, is a postgraduate fashion student
'Funnily enough, considering my thing is fashion, I like to see a woman in jeans and a crisp white shirt, preferably a man's. She needs to look as if she's just got out of the shower and have a silky skin. If she satisfies these criteria, I couldn't care less if she's a stone or so overweight. Thin women tend to be more neurotic anyway, and neurotic definitely *isn't* fabulous.'

ALISTAIR McLAREN, 34, is a policeman
'I think short hair's fabulous. I think good shoulders in a strapless dress are fabulous. I think the sight of a woman's back, as long as it's not flabby, is fabulous. I like a slightly sun-kissed skin, but not burnt brown. I adore a skin which smells good. Apart from that list, I'm not bothered what she does, how old she is or how tall!'

• • • • • • • • • • • • •

Your Image

What we look like is not the same as the impression we make. You can have your colours 'done', your style co-ordinated and your image analysed, but it won't necessarily make you a success if you have the wrong image for other reasons. So are such things a waste of time?

Well, yes and no. We all thrash around trying to find the right style when we're young, and our biggest mistake is wanting to look like someone else.

It seems that for some people, all the designer labels and correct colours and shapes in the world can't alter the image they portray. The lesson, of course, is to use this principle to your best advantage. If you haven't got two pennies to rub together and are struggling to look chic and sophisticated on a student grant, the remains of the housekeeping or income support, you can still portray a classy, chic image.

My late mother was a good example. Widowed young, she struggled to bring us up with just two dresses and a suit to her name, and she even mangled washing wearing high heels. People were less informal in those days, but even so the impression she gave was one of effortless elegance and sophistication. She added glamour with a brooch or string of cheap pearls, but I'm sure nobody who saw her would have thought those pearls were anything less than the real thing. On a tiny budget and two shopping trips a year she looked affluent and sophisticated, rather at odds with the depressing reality.

So how is it done?

People who are classy and elegant portray an understated, sartorially restrained appearance. It might seem politically incorrect to define people in terms of class these days, but looking classy has nothing to do with social status. Here are the general guidelines for a classy look:

● simplicity
● good posture
● not looking as if you are trying too hard
● not too much jewellery
● nails not too long
● not using clothes to impress
● clothes sitting comfortably on the body
● not too many highlights in your hair
● simple hair of one length, or not too many layers
● subtle make-up

Beauty is an entire effect

Looking beautiful and creating an image for yourself depends on tying up all the loose ends. This book is all about getting the foundations right, and creating an entire effect which cannot be spoiled. Getting your clothes right is important as it gives you confidence and makes the most of your figure, and I suggest you read Carol Spenser's great book, *Style Counsel* (Boxtree) which is full of fantastic tips. It shows how you can transform your style and make the best of your clothes simply by switching around what goes with what, so do try it.

Be realistic

If you go for a facelift, be advised that it won't bring back your erring husband, find you a handsome toyboy or get you invited to more parties. Buying new outfits should carry the same cautionary reminder. If you have your eye on someone and want to beat the opposition, a stunning new dress won't hook him. Well, it might if it's ten inches above

● ● ● ● ● ● ● ● ● ● ● ● ●

the knee and teamed with a pair of thigh-high boots, but that's a different story.

People notice what you look like –

– not necessarily what you are wearing. If you are always showered with compliments every time you wear that green silk trouser suit you bought five years ago, why go out and buy a floaty blue skirt just because it's high fashion? We all need new clothes, but take note of what suits you, build up a comprehensive wardrobe of outfits which incorporate all the best features, and refuse to be swayed by the newest fashion fad unless you're sure it's you. Knowing when you're well off is a knack worth acquiring, so take note of the effect of your outfits and ditch those which don't work.

If in doubt, don't!

My own golden rule of thumb for accessories – an extra chain, scarf or brooch – is that if I have to spend ten minutes prancing about in front of my mirror trying them this way and that way, they won't work. Accessories that are right look right instantly. If something only looks fantastic if you stand on one leg with your arm crooked and the other one in the air – rather like a dummy in a shop window – you shouldn't have bought it in the first place. If you're some way in between, it's not so bad. The good think about accessories is that they can be added or subtracted and nobody need know. Most of us have carried something a bit over-the-top in our handbags, waited to see what everyone else is wearing and then either brought it out or left it hidden.

If you look good in something, you'll always look good in it

Most of us have something which we look good in, so if it works, keep wearing it. If an occasion is unfamiliar or important to you, you won't want to be worrying about how an outfit works, so stick to what you know. Nobody ever lost her friends just because they'd seen her dress before,

• • • • • • • • • • • • •

and true confidence is having the courage to stay the same. Here's why:

- You'll know how to move, sit, stand and juggle drinks and plates in something you've worn before. A new outfit can be unexpectedly stiff, easily creased, ride up or slide off your shoulders. Only by wearing something will you discover how it works in practice.
- You won't feel self-conscious in it. Being able to forget your outfit is terribly important.
- You'll save time and money, both of which can be better spent making yourself glamorous in other ways.

I got married in a white suit I'd had for nine years. I had no time to shop, I was over forty, so a frothy concoction of lace and bows was out, and I knew how the suit worked. I could sit, stand, bend, sign the register, pose for photographs and get in and out of cars in it. I knew its little fault of riding up to show the lining if I wasn't careful. I knew the jacket could gape if I didn't undo one button when sitting in a low armchair. Yes, they were faults, but all clothes have their faults. I simply didn't have the time to spend an evening finding out the wearability faults of a whole new wedding outfit.

Try to buy clothes when you don't have anything special in mind and you can devote a day to the search. If you're not desperate you won't mind coming home with nothing, and you'll save money.

Always carry 'spares'

It always amazes me when people go out for a whole day taking a silly little handbag with room for no more than a lipstick, comb and the tube fare home. If you ladder your stocking or your zip breaks or you lose the back of your earring, the party's over. The 'Famous Disasters' section (see pages 166–70) gives real-life stories of disasters which couldn't have been prevented, but which we can all learn from. You don't want to embark on a fun day out with a suitcase which looks as though you're off for a fortnight in the Caribbean, but carrying a sensible emergency kit with spare tights, plasters, earring backs, hairgrips and slides, wet wipes and powder seems like basic common sense.

• • • • • • • • • • • • •

Keeping Up Appearances

Shattering the illusion

It pays to remember that however much effort you put into your appearance, it's a shame if you spoil the effect with something offputting. I don't need to mention the obvious, such as stubbing out your cigarette in your pudding or yelling a four-letter word, but people still do it!

Whether or not you choose to swear like a trooper in public is up to you, but don't be surprised if someone takes exception. It would be a miserable old world if we all went about minding our p's and q's and never saying anything either controversial or shocking, but there's a limit. The limit is when you either upset or offend someone, or you adversely affect your own chances, be they romantic, professional or social. If you're truly among friends who take you as they find you, indiscretions are usually forgiven and forgotten. Remember, though, that some people are friendly but not friends, and have no loyalty to you to keep quiet if they sense a good story at your expense.

Think of the future

You can't spend your life keeping tight-lipped just in case you might feel like standing for Parliament in twenty years' time. Worrying about every off-the-cuff remark in case you're drinking with a future employer, or living in fear of a mild profanity in case that gorgeous hunk happens to be the local vicar, is going a bit far. But don't dismiss such cautionary tales out of hand. Depending on where you are on the ladder of life, these things could matter a lot. It takes only a split second to ruin a reputation. A friend who, ten years ago, got drunk at the office Christmas party and lifted her sweater, shouting at the boss, 'What d'you think of that then?' was rewarded with his honest opinion: she wasn't promoted.

When you are young, it's great to be different from the crowd and it's nice to be noticed and talked about. The trouble is, people's memories are long when it comes to a major social gaffe, and living it down can become a problem. Do remember that if you liven up some tedious and dull social occasion with your bad behaviour it may then be talked about for years afterwards. Some people even have trouble being taken seriously again. Most problems are fuelled by alcohol, so if you can't hold your drink, don't start. You might get away with a tactless remark, but if you strip naked and seduce your host in front of his wife, you might as well emigrate.

Don't be tongue-tied

It's awful being shy, but knowing that your appearance is spot-on gives you confidence, so work on it. Generally speaking, shy people worry about what to say at parties, thinking that they haven't an opinion. It isn't like that. Ask *other people* the questions, and remember that we're all human beings who have a lot in common. Let's face it, where would we all be if it wasn't for the good old British weather, stalwart prop of 50 per cent of all conversations?

Tips to improve your image

This is so easy, you'll wonder why you wasted all that money on clothes.

- Smile as much as you can. Smile the minute you enter a room, however nervous you are. If it doesn't come naturally, practise at home in your bedroom until you get it right. Borrow a camcorder if possible and watch yourself. Coming into a room with a worried expression shows you up as self-conscious and unsure.

- Stand up straight (see 'What about body language', page 24).
- Listen attentively to the person you're speaking to. However tempted you may be, don't look over their shoulder, even for a second.
- Remember people's names. They'll be flattered and like you all the more.
- Look interested. People aren't looking to you to entertain them, but by appearing interested in others you will draw them to you. However daunting someone seems, perhaps as a captain of industry or the third richest person in England or a TV soap opera star, they still have home lives like the rest of us. An old college friend of mine who became a household name on television once lamented that at parties people never asked about her work, or commented on it. Remember, most people like being asked questions about their lives.
- Don't fiddle with handbag, jewellery or hair. It looks self-conscious and nervous and you might come across as troubled or hard work.
- If you receive a compliment, accept it with a 'Thank you'. Far too many women devalue a compliment by arguing against it.
- Work on your voice if you're worried about it. Many an illusion is shattered the minute someone opens his or her mouth.

Keep a bit back for later

I've spoken to hundreds of men about what shattered their illusions about someone or put them off. 'Keeping a bit back for another time' was high on the list. Remember that if you start at the top, the only place to go is down, so if you tell your best jokes, dazzle everyone with your stunning beauty, fantastic dancing and the amazing story of your life, you won't have the same appeal when you run into someone in the supermarket on a wet Saturday afternoon. It isn't so bad if you're in familiar company and everyone knows you, but don't go the whole hog among strangers.

Mystery is important. However extrovert you are, however effervescent and bubbly and full of life – keep a bit back for next time.

Never underestimate 'scarcity value'

When there's rumour of an imminent shortage of something, everyone wants it. The same goes for people. However, 'scarcity value' isn't to be confused with 'playing hard to get', that tedious game which wins you no friends and gets you a reputation as haughty and hard work; it is a genuine incentive to men to try that bit harder to win you.

The trick is to be bright, breezy and not too available. You don't need to go as far as I once did, and write yourself a dozen unlikely invitation cards to prop up on your mantelpiece the minute Mr Wonderful drops by, or have all your friends call you just to ensure your phone is buzzing non-stop. Being unavailable means you can't get a babysitter, your exams are looming or you can't get a night off from work. The old hair-washing routine always worked a treat, because when a man thinks that your hair is more important than him, he'll try even harder. Being a bit scarce means that by the time you say 'yes', he'll be a nervous wreck that you'll turn him down again – but won't have given up yet. And when you do say yes, he won't be taking you for granted.

What is your face saying?

If people keep on telling you to 'Cheer-up – it might never happen', take it seriously. You might be having a whale of a time or be concentrating on the finer points of someone's story, but what is your face saying?

Nobody wants to get stuck with someone who looks like hard work, and if they sense that they're going to be treated to an hour's lecture on the unfairness of the child-support system or the dog's life your ex-husband gave you, they're not even going to start.

Study yourself. Make a pleasant face which is 'lifted' without actually smiling. Think of something nice which brings a slight sparkle to your eyes, lift your eyebrows just a little. Think LIFT. Remember how it feels, and while you are training yourself, put a mirror nearby which you can keep checking.

All these things – your voice, your expression and your posture – are matters of habit. If you can get into bad habits you can also get into good ones.

What about body language?

It's time we thought about posture. No matter what you put on your back or how much money you spend beautifying, a hunched, slouched appearance destroys the whole effect.

In case you think that a straight back is all right for formal occasions but not so appropriate at casual events, I'm going to show you that you can look relaxed and confident even when perched on a sofa in a pair of jeans and a sweater. Confidence is all about good posture, so let's start with the basics:

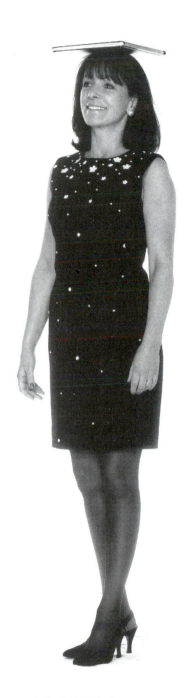

Place a large but not too heavy book on the top of your head. Move it about until it feels comfortable and won't fall off.

Walk around the room, remembering to relax your shoulders. See yourself in a full-length mirror. You might feel that your chin is too high and you are looking up. You aren't. Your chest might also feel thrust out. It isn't. Look at yourself, walk around the room again and remember what it feels like.

Practise this posture move for a few minutes twice a day, until you get used to it. Good posture is youthful. Good posture spells confidence. Practice makes perfect.

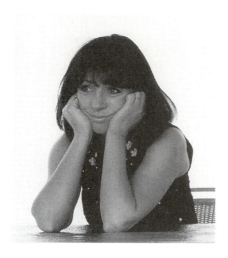

This sitting position (left), is very common, especially when it's late and you are tired, or you've had a bit too much to drink!

The second picture (below) may look a little formal, but you are still leaning on the table in a relaxed way. By keeping your back straight you look alert and interested in what people have to say, all of which gains you bonus points. It is especially important to maintain

an alert bearing if you are attending a company or business function, because even if your attitude and performance are not actually being assessed, it might be unconsciously noted that your professional bearing can slip, or was not natural.

In the first picture, by cupping your chin in this way you are not only forcing your mouth into an unattractive line, you are distorting your cheek and probably smudging your make-up. The hunched position will also leave your neck and shoulders tense.

Sit up straight, bring your chair nearer to the table, and feel the lower part of your back in contact with it. By practising now, sitting up straight will come to you naturally in the future.

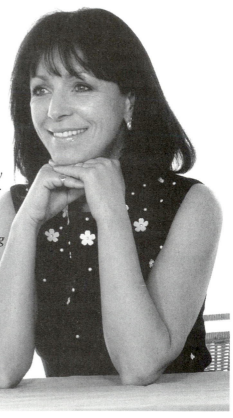

• • • • • • • • • • • • •

These two pictures speak for themselves.

If you're sitting for hours at a party and are absorbed by the conversation, it's easy to adopt the first pose (right). By raising your upper chest, the effect is far more pleasing.

Again, below, you can look relaxed but not sloppy. Note that the neck is lengthened, not hunched.

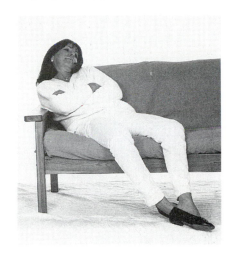

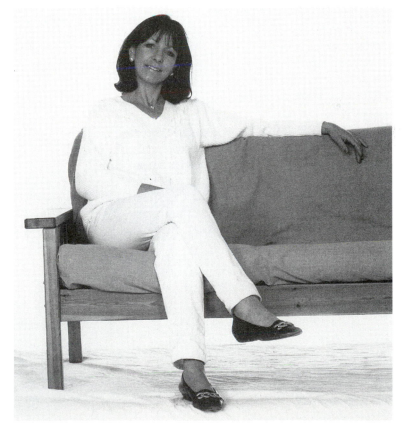

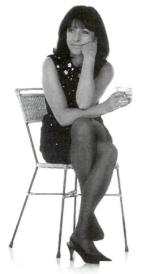

Sitting with your legs coiled round each other spoils their line. If you are uneasy about your legs, crossing them doesn't help. Your whole body line needs straightening to avoid tummy bulge and chest droop.

This sitting position (below) still looks relaxed. Try sliding your bottom right to the back of the chair until you feel it touch your back. Arch your back very slightly to its natural curve and incline

yourself forward from the waist. Cross your legs at the ankles and not knees, to avoid bulging thighs.

Placing your spare hand on your leg might feel awkward, but it looks quite relaxed and natural. Try it, and get used to how it feels.

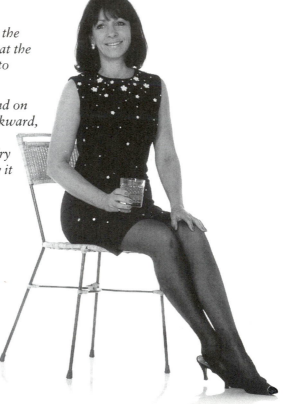

The Diet

You can't look good if you don't eat. Nor can you look good if you eat rubbish. Your hair, skin, nails and even your moods all depend on good nourishment. A deficient diet can significantly alter your moods and lead to depression, and if you're going to look good you have to feel good.

We get fat because we eat too much. No surprises there. We also eat chaotically, which means grabbing food on the run, eating in the street, eating at our desks, eating at any time of the day and night. Then when we want to lose weight we cut out meals and go hungry. Wrong. To lose weight you must eat smaller amounts more often, eat breakfast, eat more starch and get more exercise. And most important of all, you must discipline yourself to set meal-times, and stick to them.

The mistake people make when they see the needle on the scales shoot up is to panic, then crash into reverse gear and eat next to nothing for the following few days. It isn't necessary to be so drastic. You might think that the less you eat the quicker you'll lose weight, but it isn't like that. You only have to eat a little less and exercise a little more and your weight will start to fall. The section on metabolism (see page 46) explains this in greater detail.

Whenever I've given women my diet plan they've always commented after a few days that a) they seem to be eating a lot more and b) they don't feel as if they're on a diet. We somehow feel that we should be suffering in order to lose weight, but this isn't necessary. You don't even have to give up any of your favourite foods. The only banned foods are those which are either addictive, such as chocolate and coffee, or bad for your looks, as in the case of fried foods, sweets and fizzy colas.

A fresh start

This is a makeover diet. You don't have to be getting married or taking the holiday of a lifetime. If you are choosing this plan simply to lose a few pounds and look better, you will.

In my book *5 Days to a Flatter Stomach*, I told you how to achieve a flatter stomach not just by losing weight, but by avoiding certain types and combinations of food which encourage bloating and leave you hungry. I am sticking with the same principles for your fortnight's plan because I believe in them, the only slight variations being in the amount of fruit you can eat in the daytime, and the inclusion of more pulse vegetables. This diet will be like a spring-clean for your system. However much you feel you've abused your diet in the past, however much you feel you're a lost cause, it's never too late to take hold of yourself, turn yourself around and make a fresh start.

The Rules

This diet is not intended to last for ever. You follow it for six days, have the seventh day off, and resume the diet for a further seven days. You then use the diet and its principles every time you want to get back on the strait and narrow after a binge, holiday or Christmas. Or you can keep to the diet for, say, weekdays only. The basic rules are these:

1. You must eat breakfast.
2. You should try to eat your main meal at lunchtime.
3. You should eat a small snack at bedtime.

• • • • • • • • • • • • • •

4. No alcohol.
5. Only decaffeinated coffee.
6. No chocolate.
7. No artificial sweeteners or diet colas.
8. One main meal with potatoes, rice or pasta every day.
9. Four pieces of fruit a day.
10. Three slices of bread a day.
11. An 'allowance' of no more than 7 g/¼ oz butter per day.
12. A pint of skimmed milk a day PLUS one glass of full-cream milk.
13. SIX glasses of water every day – in addition to other drinks.
14. One salad meal every day.

It is a restrictive diet for these reasons:

● You only have to buy a limited list of foods.
● You don't have too many choices to worry about.
● Its purpose is to improve your looks as well as your figure.

Main meals

All main meals should be accompanied by vegetables and potatoes or rice. Some meals will be pasta-based. Even if you choose a curry, a chilli or stir-fry meal, have a side plate of fresh vegetables which should include some dark, leafy ones such as cabbage, broccoli, cauliflower, spinach, etc.

Light meals

There are two or three light meal choices for each day, and even if you have chosen a toast meal, such as scrambled eggs or beans on toast, I would like you to have a side salad.

It is important that you have a salad meal every day, so if you make your own light meal to take to work, choose either a salad-based meal or sandwiches which include salad vegetables.

Plenty of variety

The days when a salad consisted of little more than limp lettuce, a few slices of cucumber and a sliced tomato are well over. Supermarkets are now full of the most varied and wonderful displays of fruit and vegetables, and we are far more experimental these days than we used to be when it comes to mixing weird and exotic ingredients in a bowl and calling it a salad.

See how many varieties of lettuce there are on the market! You can choose from cos, iceberg, feuille de chêne, lollo rosso and radicchio, not to mention lamb's lettuce and rocket, which are not true lettuces but are used as such.

Not all the recipes are lettuce-based. To help you find something different every day, the recipe section contains salads which are meat-based, fish-based, vegetarian and the newer and most popular 'warm' salads. You can have salads with fruit, nuts, cheese, grains and pulses. In fact, I know there's something to please every taste, and I'd like you to choose at least one salad from the list every day.

Restricted meat

In this diet meat is restricted to chicken. Although I am not a vegetarian myself, I hardly ever eat meat. I simply find it takes a long time to prepare and digest, and whenever I'm on an improvement plan I cut it out in favour of fish.

I have included chicken for people who find it hard to do without some kind of meat base, and indeed you can't really beat roast chicken and vegetables as a tasty meal. However, you'll notice a predominance of salmon and cod dishes, plus vegetables, salads and fruit. Anyone wanting to look her best will find this type of diet ideal.

Puddings and sweets

I have also tried to be inventive with your pudding choices, and each main meal is followed by a pudding. Your light meal should finish with fresh fruit or a bowl of fresh fruit salad.

• • • • • • • • • • • • • •

Never neglect your milk

I fear for future generations of women, especially those brought up in diet-conscious families. Too much fat is definitely bad for you, but we've cut out full-fat milk to a worrying degree, and I truly believe in milk as a beauty aid. Not only does it keep your skin looking good, it guards against osteoporosis in later life as it contains calcium, protein and vitamins. Try to drink a glass of full-cream milk every day, in addition to your skimmed milk. If you have plenty of milk and water in your diet, you won't go far wrong. Although it's a bore to think about health when you're young, believe me, it's worth it. I can't say I really enjoy drinking a glass of milk, but that's not the point. Get it down you and reap the benefits.

Spelling it out

It was a hard decision, but I wanted to spell out your meals for you simply to avoid giving you an impossibly long list of alternatives. Too much choice is stressful, and your main priorities in the next fortnight are to work on your looks and figure. If the meals for any day don't suit you, choose from another day. I have calorie-counted each day's meals, so you won't exceed your limit, whichever day you choose from.

You might find these rules hard to stick with, but that is because most people have become used to an undisciplined way of eating. We also drink too much alcochol, which not only piles on the weight, it makes you lose your resolve not to pig out. These are the reasons people have weight problems. 'I don't want to eat my main meal at lunchtime,' they say, or 'I find it impossible to eat breakfast.' But they can't lose weight. Fine, but if your old way isn't working, why stick with it? Isn't it worth trying something different just for a fortnight?

I can make you these promises while you are on my Fabulous in a Fortnight plan:

• • • • • • • • • • • • •

1. You WILL lose weight, and with the exercises you will IMPROVE your shape.
2. You will have much more energy.
3. You will sleep well.
4. Your skin will start to improve.

More than just weight loss

This diet is about more than just losing weight. We can all weigh less and look just as bad as we did before, only skinnier. Weighing less says nothing about how you LOOK, so this diet is also aimed at the quality of food you are putting inside yourself. Diets of fruit, salad and grilled fish are highly nutritious and you'll lose weight on them, but if you don't eat carbohydrates you'll feel washed out and feeble. Such diets leave you so tired you can't do your exercise, which rather defeats the object. Looking fabulous means looking not just slim but bright, bouncy, cheerful and healthy, and on this diet you'll feel all of this and more. More? Yes, you'll also feel confident.

So no fattening foods?

Food is not fattening. Food is just fuel. It's like saying that a car is dangerous. A car can't do anything by itself except sit there, and it's only when we get in it that it becomes potentially dangerous. Food doesn't turn to fat the minute we swallow it. Some foods contain more calories per gram than others, but that's another thing. Anything you eat too much of – be it fish or apples or rice – will make you fat, but it's all down to you in the end.

What's this about sleepless nights?

It isn't true to say that eating late makes you gain weight. Plenty of people such as professional dancers and actors have to eat late because of their work, and don't gain weight. Lots of people stop eating after their evening meal and are still fat. What you have to watch, though, is eating meat, fried food and heavy puddings late, especially if you have been sitting all evening. Eating after exercise is a brilliant way to eat because it's like putting cotton wool into a furnace, so it's best to go out to a good exercise class or sports activity on a relatively empty stomach, and eat afterwards. Your metabolism stays high for a couple of hours after *vigorous* exercise, and your food is burnt up more efficiently. I shall talk more about this in the exercise section of the book.

It is wise to have a starchy snack before bedtime, to prevent midnight raids on the fridge. I have suggested a small bowl of porridge, or a slice of toast, both of which are light on the stomach and easily digested. I have had a porridge supper every night for the past twenty years!

Eating early, say before six o'clock in the evening, means that by three in the morning it is nine hours since you last ate and your blood sugar could be low. This wakes you up. Most of us are familiar with the syndrome, when we feel so bright that we get up and do the washing! The downside is that we get back to sleep only to wake at the usual time feeling as if we have a hangover. This is classic low-blood sugar. A starchy breakfast such as cereal or toast will bring you back nicely and you will start to feel alert, but unfortunately the sort of people who suffer in this way also tend not to be breakfast eaters. EVERYBODY should eat breakfast, however. It is common sense, and I have noticed that most people with weight problems say they skip breakfast.

NOTE: *If you continue to sleep badly after amending your eating pattern, it's wise to see your doctor. Other conditions and hormonal disturbances can also cause sleeplessness.*

How will my skin improve?

Fortunately, the length of this diet means that your skin has a chance to improve. Skin renews itself every three to five days, depending on your age, and although it won't work immediately, I can promise you that if you follow all the beauty routines, drink plenty of water and eat the diet as prescribed, you will see a significant improvement in your skin in a fortnight.

This diet works. Once you embrace the idea of a change in your way of eating, you'll be well on your way!

• • • • • • • • • • • • • •

Good Nutrition

The main ingredients of this diet are potatoes and rice. The next most important foods are fruit, fish, milk, vegetables and bread. In smaller quantities you'll have pasta and chicken. The idea is that you eat the diet for six days, and relax on the seventh.

I have deliberately kept to a limited list of foods to make shopping easier, and so that you don't have too many choices or uneaten foods in the fridge! Most people like potatoes in one form or another, they are extremely cheap and can be made into a variety of dishes. I have chosen other foods which can be eaten raw, or which take the minimum of cooking. However much you might like cooking – and some of you love to experiment, I know – it's important that you get out of the kitchen in the next fortnight and spend more time exercising and attending to your face, hair and body. So *no excuses* about being too busy in the kitchen!

How much do I need?

There's a lot of talk about what proportion of a certain nutrient we need in our diet, but how on earth do we know what 70 per cent means in terms of slices of bread, or 30 per cent when it comes to our intake of eggs or chicken? Basically, what is a really healthy diet?

Complex carbohydrates

You should take about 70 per cent of your food in the form of carbohydrates. Carbohydrates are not stodgy or fattening, they are essential for fuel. During exercise, your muscles are fuelled by glucose in the blood, and by glycogen, which is stored in your liver and muscles. Muscles normally contain enough glycogen to fuel between one and two hours of vigorous exercise.

Potatoes, rice and bread contain complex carbohydrate which releases its energy over a prolonged period and therefore decreases the likelihood of hunger pangs or cravings. You also get carbohydrates from fruit, vegetables, pulses and pasta.

Here are some typical combinations which contain mostly complex carbohydrates and some simple sugars. They would be enough for one day:

50 g/2 oz breakfast cereal	*or* 1 bowl cornflakes
4 large slices bread	1 helping pasta
175 g/6 oz boiled potatoes	2 small bunches grapes
1 pear	1 orange
1 peach	mixed bean salad
1 scone	3 slices bread
	or 1 packet crisps
	1 jacket potato
	2 bananas
	1 apple
	1 digestive biscuit
	2 large slices bread

NOTE: *The durum wheat used to make pasta is hard and high in gluten, which many people cannot tolerate. If you suffer from irritable bowels or wheat intolerance, I suggest you eat less pasta and more potatoes and rice, with plenty of fruit. Coeliac disease is very serious and sufferers cannot tolerate gluten. However, many people simply find certain cereals cause bloating and dis-*

comfort, so the following list of foods which either contain gluten or not might be useful.

WITH GLUTEN
Barley
Oats
Semolina
Rye
Wheat

GLUTEN-FREE
Maize (as in popcorn, cornflour)
Rice
Millet

Proteins

Proteins are necessary for the formation and maintenance of body tissues.

Eating too much protein in the belief that it will be beneficial to health is not only a waste of time, it can actually be harmful. Protein cannot be stored in the body so the excess is converted in the liver to glucose. A by-product is urea which must be excreted. This makes your urine acidic, which in turn leads to loss of calcium from the bones. In previous centuries, when a diet high in massive quantities of meat was commonplace, bone weakening was a sympton.

Despite the relative gluttony of many athletes, who regularly eat up to ten egg whites a day and consume huge quantities of meat in their attempts to build their muscles, surplus protein is not stored as muscle. The nitrogen is removed and excreted, and the remainder is used for energy or stored as glycogen or fat. No harm comes from eating rather more protein than your daily requirement on occasion, but don't make it a habit. An eventual weight gain is inevitable, however, from an excessive calorie intake from any source, and just because your food is fat-free or 'healthy' does not mean that you will not gain weight if you eat too much of it.

How much protein you need in one day

An average man needs around 50 g/2 oz of protein a day, the average woman needs about 45 g/1½ oz. This can be derived from the following foods:

225 g/8 oz roast chicken
250 g/9 oz poached or grilled fish
25 g/1 oz nuts
6 slices bread

Remember, too, that many other foods contain protein, such as pasta, milk, cheese and eggs, and it is extremely unlikely that any Western diet would be deficient, as requirements are modest.

Fats

Views on fat intake in the diet have changed enormously over the past thirty years, and there is still a debate about how much fat is good for you. One thing is certain: a diet which contains no fat at all is an extremely bad and dangerous one. We need fat for the absorption of certain vitamins, and it is important to our skin, hair, nails and general health. We all know that intakes of saturated fat are linked with heart disease: as a guide, a saturated fat is one which hardens at room temperature, such as butter and lard, and they tend to be of animal origin.

The subject is a wide one, and if you would like to know more, I suggest you read *The Fats We Need to Eat* by Jeanette Ewin (Thorsons).

How much fat you need in one day

You need around 25 g/1 oz of fat a day for the body to absorb fat-soluble vitamins. The best way to calculate your 25 g is to read food information labels on bought products.

Omega-3 fatty acids are needed in small amounts, and can be found in the following:

a handful of walnuts
a 100 g/4 oz oily fish such as mackerel
2 teaspoonfuls vegetable oil (as in a salad dressing)

• • • • • • • • • • • • •

Omega-6 fatty acids, found in nuts, seeds and polyunsaturated oils, are needed in similar amounts.

Fats can also be obtained from avocado pears, dairy products and meat.

Remember that eating fatless dishes such as a fatless sponge cake, meringues or boiled rice, can still put on weight if you eat too much of them. None of these foods contains fat, but consuming half a dozen meringues, a whole sponge cake or several plates of rice just because they are fatless won't do your weight any favours!

If you could only eat three foods, what would they be?

Opinions vary on this. In purely health terms my choice would be bananas, carrots and nuts. Bananas give you carbohydrate and fibre, carrots provide betacarotene, fibre and water, and nuts contain protein and fat. A balanced choice.

Vitamins and minerals

People often ask about vitamin supplements when they are feeling run down, tired or depressed.

First, I want to get one problem out of the way because it is something I am asked about every week by slimmers who are struggling to achieve their goal weight, only to find themselves looking and feeling awful, with puffy eyes and a debilitating lethargy. I talk about this a lot because I feel strongly about it. It seems to me to defeat the object completely if you strive to look good, then feel so washed out that all you can do is curl up on the sofa in your nightie and watch the box.

As I am a complete believer in eating plenty, eating frequently and eating carbohydrate-rich foods which give you energy, I am always confident that my clients are not suffering from lack of proper nourishment, which is obviously a reason to feel lethargic. There are two other causes of tiredness which are not necessarily related to diet, and those are stress and boredom. Feeling tired doesn't always mean that you need sleep. Many workaholics manage on very few hours' sleep a night; they have their work to keep them bright and on top of the world. By contrast, having a monotonous and repetitive life can spell boredom, not to be confused with having nothing to do. Many people who feel tired all the time go to the chemist's and stock up on vitamin pills and tonics, when in fact a dull or uninteresting life is the cause.

Stress is also very draining and can make you feel 'heady', as if you are suffering from flu. Sufferers usually find that a change of scene or some brisk exercise does the trick – suddenly a new lease of life has been found! So recognize these two problems before you reach for the tablets or telephone the doctor, and try these self-help remedies:

● Eat a good breakfast with plenty of carbohydrate.
● Eat more starch, and do not go for more than three hours without food.
● Take some brisk exercise.
● Drink a pint of fresh water – dehydration makes you weak.

Remember: if your symptoms persist, see your doctor for a check-up.

A good diet is a balanced diet, and that means a bit of everything. Supplements are needed if you are a smoker, if you exercise a lot, or do a job which is physically demanding. Our daily iron requirement is 14mg, which is the dose found in most standard iron preparations. I suggest you take a combined multivitamin with iron tablet every day, as iron is lost through perspiration, and the extra minerals, especially potassium, will also help. Loss of potassium and salt causes cramping, and loss of fluid generally makes you feel very weak. It is not generally understood just how great an effect lack of fluid can have on your alertness. Everybody should drink at least two litres of fluid every day, and eat food which has a high water content, like fruit and vegetables.

● ● ● ● ● ● ● ● ● ● ● ● ● ●

Free radicals and anti-oxidants

We hear a lot of talk of 'free-radicals' these days. Skin creams tell us they contain anti-oxidants to defend the body against free radicals, certain vitamins are said to help the body fight free radical attack, and so forth. But many people do not understand exactly what free radicals are, so I have included a brief explanation here.

Research into free radicals is in its infancy, which is why we haven't heard much about them until recently. The technology needed to look into the question simply wasn't available until about ten years ago, a short time in medical research terms. But free radicals are something we all ought to be concerned about, especially when we are thinking of our looks, the ageing process and our health.

The body is made up of tissues and cells. These cells are made up of molecules. Within the molecules are electrons, and electrons like to go around in pairs.

A free radical is a molecule with an unpaired electron. It therefore sets about trying to find another electron to pair with, and when it finds one, it leaves another electron without a partner, and so on. This continual search for a pair leads to a cascade of reactions, and this in turn leads to cell damage and damage to the body.

Free radicals start their journey of destruction because the body's cells are being attacked by poisons from food and the atmosphere. Indeed, two of our worst enemies are sunlight and tobacco smoke, which trigger free radicals and cause the skin ageing we associate with both smoking and sun damage, as well as related cancers.

However, just as the body is able to ward off infections and illnesses, it is also brilliantly designed to take on free radical attack by the production of anti-oxidant defences. These primarily take the form of vitamins E and C. If we are at risk from enhanced radical attack – perhaps because we live in a polluted environment, if we smoke cigarettes or suffer from passive smoking, or expose ourselves to the sun – the body's normal defences may not be enough. Therefore, to prevent free radical attack we should either take vitamin supplements, or, better still, eat a diet which includes plenty of foods rich in anti-oxidants.

Vitamins which guard against free radicals:

VITAMIN A and BETACAROTENE

Vitamin A is present in liver, dairy produce and oily fish. Betacarotene is an especially valuable anti-oxidant, and is responsible for the colour in vegetables such as red and yellow peppers and carrots.

VITAMIN E

Vitamin E stimulates our immune response, and should be taken by people on low-cholesterol diets who over-consume polyunsaturated oils. Found in nuts, seeds, fish oils, seeds and wheatgerm. You do not need much of this vitamin – a handful of nuts a day or the addition of a tablespoonful of wheatgerm to a dish is quite sufficient.

VITAMIN C

Found in all citrus fruits, cranberries, kiwifruit, potatoes and vegetables such as peppers.

SELENIUM

The trace mineral selenium is a powerful protector against free radicals and cancer. Butter, brazil nuts, avocados, lentils and shellfish are particularly rich in selenium.

NOTE: *On this diet plan, you should not need more than one multivitamin and iron tablet a day. The diet is worked out to provide you with everything you need for energy and glowing looks.*

On each day on the fortnight's plan, you will be given a choice of meals with their calorie content. I expect you to lose between five and seven pounds in weight, depending on the weight you started at. The main thing to remember, however, is to note how you *look*. Having a low weight is no guarantee of a good shape, so don't get too hung up by what the scales say. Just stick to the diet, and see the difference in your energy, skin and clothes size. You won't be disappointed!

The importance of water

I cannot stress enough how important it is to take plenty of fluid. Yes, but I forget to drink! one woman said to me recently. Or, 'I don't want to be going to the loo all the time,' said another. Oh dear. I'm afraid that when it comes to drinking water – not the most exciting drink – you have to view it like taking your medicine, brushing your teeth or having your hair colour sorted out. Not the most pleasant thing in the world, but a matter of routine, with results which are worth it.

Water is valuable to us in several ways:

1. It helps ease the passage of food through the gut, and is therefore vital to a flat stomach.
2. It helps flush the system of poisons which cause spotty skins.
3. It helps 'plump out' your skin, to avoid a dried-prune appearance.

Your food also contains a lot of water, so if you regularly follow a controlled diet and eat only one main meal a day, you will also be lacking in fluid and should drink extra. Two signs of not drinking enough are a blinding headache and lassitude.

NOTE: *On the Fabulous in a Fortnight plan, you will be drinking an EXTRA six glasses (150 ml/15 fl oz each) of water every day.*

• • • • • • • • • • • • •

A Question of Metabolism

I couldn't write a book about diet and not mention metabolism. Most of my clients bring up the subject when they have reached a plateau in their diet, their complaint being that they're eating very little and not losing any more weight. Clients who have been cutting back too drastically on their food and then start to eat normally find their weight rises. 'I promise you I'm not eating more than 1,500 calories a day!' they cry, and I believe them. A thyroid problem is often suspected, but although I always recommend that they see their doctor if they're seriously worried, I know that their problem is low metabolism from eating too little.

It sorts itself out

When you've been dieting you have to go back to normal eating habits at some stage. You can't be on a diet all your life, but you can formulate a realistic diet for the rest of your life which takes your lifestyle into account. When you've been cutting back on food, a slight weight rise is inevitable once you start to re-introduce more food. Most of the weight gain is fluid. You must remember that to gain a pound of fat you would have to eat an *extra* 3,500 calories in a short space of time, so if you know that you are eating sensibly, sit tight. The weight rise will go back down again as soon as your body has adjusted.

The human body works on a principle called *homeostasis*, its ability to regulate itself over weeks and months rather than hours or days. This is why short periods without food, such as during a brief crisis or extra workload, will not have a lasting effect on your weight, nor will a short period of overeating, such as a heavy weekend away or a few days when you eat yourself out of house and home. As long as you go back to your normal eating habits, the body will adjust very quickly.

What is the metabolic rate?

The metabolic rate is the rate at which your body burns its fuel. It's like the difference between a Rolls-Royce and a Mini. Strangely enough, the fatter a person is, the higher the rate at which they burn calories, simply because it takes a lot of effort to move a larger person around. What you might not realize is that you can change your metabolic rate, higher or lower, in about a week or two, and eating less actually slows down your rate.

Sorting fact from fiction

Your body needs fuel, even if you lie in bed and do nothing. Your basic metabolic rate is around 1,450 calories for a woman and 1,900 for a man, and the mistake we make is in thinking that food is fuel which has to be 'burned off'. True, food is our fuel, but it is needed for your energy stores so that if you have stressful times when you have to spend a fraught day without eating, you can still function. I'm not talking about fat stores. They're extra. I'm talking about stores of glycogen in the muscles, without which we'd feel constantly tired, lethargic and unable to move. You don't put food in and instantly burn it off.

So how do I raise my metabolism?

You raise your metabolism through exercise which increases your proportion of muscle to fat, through regular aerobic exercise and regular food intake. It works like this.

The greater your proportion of muscle to fat, the higher your metabolism. Your weight tells you nothing about your body compositon. Rather like the difference between a pound of butter and a pound of feathers, you can weigh nine stone of flabby, fatty flesh or nine stone of well-toned, taut muscle. The less fat you have, the more you can eat to stay the same weight because muscle is 'living'. Muscles do a job. Muscles have a blood supply and have to move your bones. They get hot and can stretch and contract. Every movement you make requires muscles, and servicing muscle requires a high metabolism. If you increase your muscle content you will be able to eat more food.

Fat does nothing at all. It sits there as your emergency food supply. The body lets us put on fat to enable us to stay alive if we are in danger of starvation. In fact, your body wants you to stay alive until the last possible moment, so it has this wonderful way of helping you to store fat, and when you starve yourself it will not only save fat, but will consume your muscles and any other stores it can get hold of, such as calcium from your bones. If you diet too stringently, you will not be aware of what your body is doing to you, the only warning signs being tiredness. You will be feeling euphoric because you are thin, but your body is struggling. Your metabolic rate will be falling as your body sets into panic mode, and you'll be trying on size 8s. Eventually, you either decide to eat again, or you give in to hunger and binge. Whichever way, you will gain weight very quickly.

NOTE: *Keep your metabolic rate high by eating regularly, eating carbohydrate, and exercising every day.*

The key is regularity

The only way to raise your metabolic rate and keep it high, so that you can eat more some days and less on others *and not affect your weight* is to be regular in your habits of eating and exercising.

Don't go to the gym only when you have had a heavy weekend bingeing. You won't work it off like that. Get into

• • • • • • • • • • • • • •

regular habits which suit your lifestyle, such as three sessions a week of keep-fit, a morning walk on Tuesdays, Thursdays and Saturdays and some toning exercises for your muscles which are done a couple of times a day. Little and often. Three five-minute stomach tightening sessions a day are better than one manic session, and you're less likely to get bored or injured.

It's the same with food. 'But you told me to eat less to get slim, now you're saying eat more!' is another frequent complaint. No, you eat more OFTEN, not more food. Split up your meals. Put out a plateful and literally halve it, saving the second half for two hours later. This may sound strange and is not a recommended course of action for the rest of your life, but to train yourself to eat smaller portions more frequently, this is what you must do. It works. Your body will trust you and not store food as fat the moment you eat, you won't get hungry, so the temptation to binge will vanish, and the weight will start to go.

So no alteration in what I eat?

I didn't say that! If you're usually a sensible, healthy eater, you only need alter the size of portions and the frequency of eating. If you have a weight problem you'll have been eating too much for your requirements at some stage, so eating smaller amounts is vital. Cutting out alcohol also helps, as we get a lot of useless calories from it. If you find that hard, you must try. Alcohol does you no good whatever, so until you have your weight under control, give it up or cut down.

If you've been eating a lot of rubbish, your eating habits will have to alter drastically if you're going to lose weight. But you can still have proper tasty food. Again, the principles are smaller portions, more frequently, and the only banned foods are those which ruin your looks or health, such as sweets, coffee, alcohol and chocolate.

• • • • • • • • • • • • •

The Exercises

Anyone under the age of about twenty-five would be for-given for thinking that exercise was introduced by Jane Fonda in the 1980s. It's common to imagine that our mothers and grandmothers only went walking or swimming, or maybe did a bit of gentle keep-fit waving a ribbon about.

In fact, the 'daily dozen', as it was called, was an essential part of every housewife's day in the 1940s and 1950s. These were exercises geared at maintaining good ankles, a trim waist and flat stomach – taken much more seriously then than I think it is today. The routines might seem sedate by today's standards, but instead of burned-out aerobics addicts, you had women who were proud of their figures, and who saw exercise as a duty to themselves and others.

Nowadays, too many women fit in exercise when they can, and plead lack of time. If this is you, *try to take a different attitude.*

No makeover plan is complete without exercising. Muscles are there to be used, and if they aren't, they become weak, the tone is lost and your body literally begins to lose its shape. You can look quite reasonable if you keep slim and don't exercise, but to look fantastic you must exercise. Exercise is essential not just for your body, but for your mind as well, and your health.

On this plan we are going to pay attention to the three main areas of exercise.

Aerobic exercise

This includes brisk walking, swimming, running and cycling. It also includes aerobic classes, which you might have near you, but if not it doesn't matter. It is just as easy to exercise briskly at home.

The reason to do aerobic exercise is to get your heart pumping and the blood flowing faster. This in turn leads to slight breathlessness and the glowing feeling you get from a really good spot of exercise. Aerobic exercise releases hormones called endorphins which are responsible for the so-called 'exercise high'.

The benefits to your circulation will show in noticeably smoother skin.

TIP: *Being short of breath while exercising can point to more than just being unfit. Lack of fluid and low iron also cause tiredness and breathlessness. See your doctor for a check-up if the problem is persistent, but try drinking more water and taking more iron-rich foods such as liver, dark leafy vegetables, egg yolks and sardines.*

Stretching exercise (flexibility)

Stretching is vital after exercise because it guards against stiffness. It helps prevent injury, too, because muscles which are short and tight become injured more quickly. Stretching is also important for the appearance of our limbs. Muscles which are gently toned, then stretched, never get big. You won't have massive thighs or calves, but you will look solid and taut, without wobble. Proper stretching takes some practice and you'll need to hold each position for a good thirty seconds, but once you notice the difference you'll want to include stretching in your daily routine for the future.

> **TIP:** *Try these tests for good flexibility: a) you should be able to put one hand down the back of your neck and place it just above and between your shoulder blades; b) lie on the floor with one leg outstretched and the calf touching the floor. Hug the other knee into your chest. You should be able to do this without your outstretched leg rising from the floor; c) bring one foot up behind you and hold it to your bottom.*

Strength exercise (toning)

This is not as bad as it sounds, and it doesn't mean that you will be lifting weights or looking like a bodybuilder. Most of the daily exercises in this book will be toning for your legs, bottom, stomach and waist, and all the exercises can be done in your own living-room or bedroom, in ten-minute sessions.

> **TIP:** *It is vital that you commit yourself to doing these exercises every day. Be sure not to overdo the exercising, especially if you are new to it. It is tempting to do too much in the belief that you will see quicker results, but it doesn't work like that, and you don't want to spend your special day encased in plaster because you've broken a leg! If in doubt about your health, see your doctor first.*

When should I eat?

Always exercise on an empty stomach, except in the case of early morning exercise, when it is a long time since your last meal. In the early morning I generally take a half-portion of porridge (15 g/½ oz of oats) if I am to exercise within an hour, but as a general rule of thumb eat *after* exercise, when your metabolism will be higher. Energy is stored in your muscles, and if you have been exercising, your energy stores will be used up. Eating after exercise puts back the lost

• • • • • • • • • • • • • •

energy supplies and feeds your existing requirements, so less is stored as fat. *Remember, though, that a heavy meal is not a good idea. Choose starch instead, and plenty of fluid.* Personally, when exercising in the evening I have a late lunch about four hours before my class. I then eat an apple as I drive home and have a light, carbohydrate-rich meal later.

It is particularly important that your stomach should be empty when you are exercising your abdomen. Abdominal exercises put great pressure on your spine and they should not be done for more than three to five minutes a time, followed by turning over and decompressing your spine by pressing it in the opposite direction.

Picture it thus: between the front and back of your body you have not only your bones, muscles and vital organs but also your stomach, intestines and their contents. Each movement in a stomach exercise forces your stomach *downwards* to your spine, and if you have a meal inside you it adds to the pressure on the disc between your vertebrae.

If you must eat something before exercise, eat a plain biscuit, slice of toast, banana or apple. Do NOT eat anything sugary. Contrary to popular belief, a bar of chocolate only gives you instant energy, and in the long term it makes you feel quite grim. The rush of sugar into the bloodstream causes a release of insulin to counter it, with the result that your blood-sugar level is lowered dramatically and you will feel washed-out and sleepy. If you happen to be exercising you will suddenly find that your arms and legs feel heavy and you can hardly lift them. It is not a pleasant feeling, and it needn't happen. Never eat a sugary or chocolatey snack on its own before exercise.

Your daily exercises

Start with a brisk walk if possible. If you go to work, have a break at lunchtime and have a walk then, whatever the weather. Sitting in the office will dull your mind and make you feel sleepy. Try not to make the excuse of having shopping to do or needing to work through your lunch hour. We all get the bodies we deserve, so getting a bit wet or leaving that report for half an hour is well worth it if you end up with a figure you can be proud of. This plan only lasts for two weeks, so make the most of it.

Daily warm-up and stretch

Every morning you should start with a wake-up stretch, which is described on Day One (see page 83).

Put on some music – I suggest something catchy with about 140 beats a minute. It might seem a bore to start finding tracks and counting beats, but it's important to get the right speed or you could either pull a muscle or take too long! The song 'I will survive' by Gloria Gaynor is about the correct speed.

• • • • • • • • • • • • •

WARM-UP
This comes in three parts – side swings, knee lifts and kick-backs:

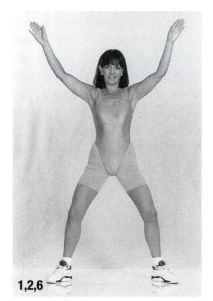

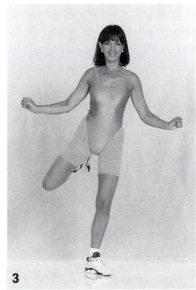

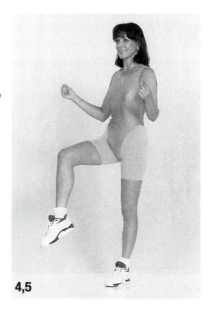

1. *Step from side to side, swinging your arms.*
2. *Do sixteen, then go into kick-backs.*
3. *Kicking each foot backwards to your bottom, and starting with arms outstretched, bring your elbows into your waist and out again. Repeat sixteen times.*
4. *Go into knee lifts.*
5. *Lift each knee as shown, doing simple elbow curls. Repeat sixteen times.*
6. *Return to side swings and repeat the sequence twice. Sixteen side swings. Sixteen kick backs. Sixteen knee lifts.*

STRETCH OUT
You have four stretches:

1. **THIGH STRETCH**
   Take each foot back towards your bottom and hold for ten seconds.

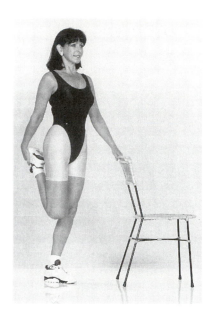

2. **HAMSTRING STRETCH**
   Resting on bent leg, stretch the back of one leg. Hold for ten seconds and change sides.

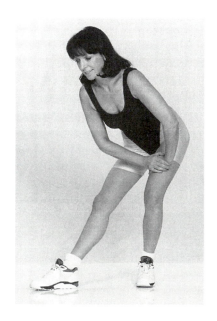

3. **CALF STRETCH**
   Follow picture, leaning slightly forwards. Change legs.

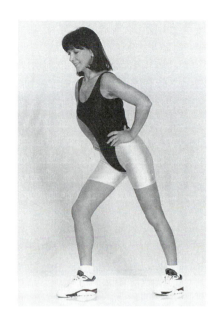

4. **SHOULDER STRETCH**
   Follow picture, holding each arm across your chest for ten seconds.

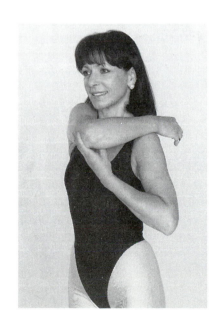

• • • • • • • • • • • • •

Muscle-toning exercises

Set aside ten to fifteen minutes for these. It isn't too much to ask of yourself if it keeps you in trim. We all frequently spend far more than twenty or thirty minutes a day just reading a magazine or newspaper or chatting, so don't begrudge the time you spend exercising.

EXERCISES FOR YOUR OUTER THIGHS

These exercises tone the outer thighs, and are especially good if you like to wear close-fitting skirts or trousers.

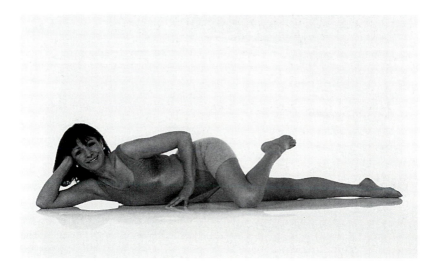

1. *Lie on your side, as shown, making sure your top hip is forward.*

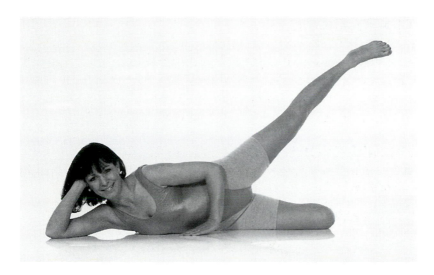

2. *Slowly extend leg to the side, taking care not to fling it.*
3. *Lower to floor again, and repeat eight times. Rest and repeat a further eight times.*

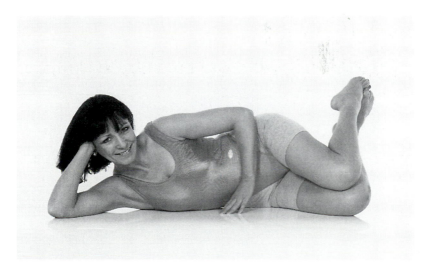

KNEE SQUEEZES
4. *Lie as shown, feet together and off the floor.*
5. *Do rapid little squeezes of the knees together. Do sixteen, rest and repeat.*

• • • • • • • • • • • • •

SIDE LEG LIFTS

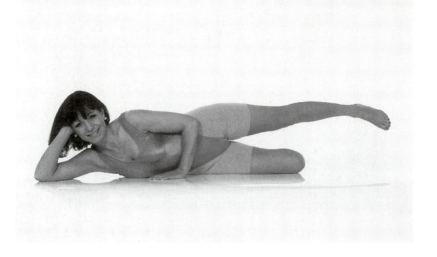

6. *With legs extended, bottom leg slightly bent, rest on one hand. Lift your top leg, being careful not to fling it upwards. Lower and raise again sixteen times (or eight if you are feeling fatigued).*

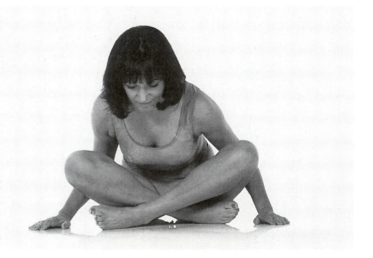

7. *With legs crossed, lean forwards and feel the stretch in your outer thighs. Hold for ten seconds. Lie on your other side and repeat the whole sequence of exercises.*

• • • • • • • • • • • • •

Exercises for your bottom

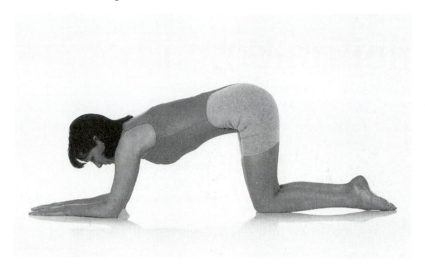

1. *Lie on all fours, elbows and knees. Keep your back straight, take the weight on your elbows, hips square to the floor and stomach pulled in tightly to support your spine.*

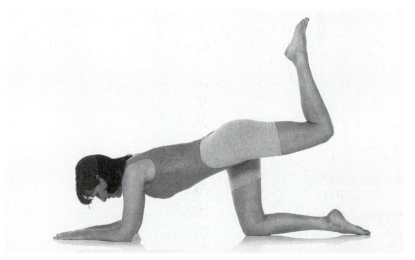

2. *Raise and lower your leg. Do sixteen, change legs and do a further sixteen.*

• • • • • • • • • • • • •

STRAIGHT LEGS RAISES

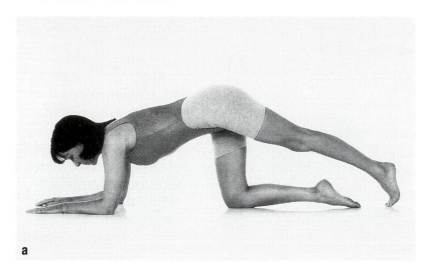

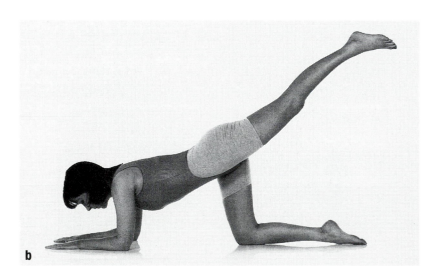

3. *Starting with one leg straight out behind you, slowly lower (a) and raise (b) eight times. Change legs and repeat.*

• • • • • • • • • • • • •

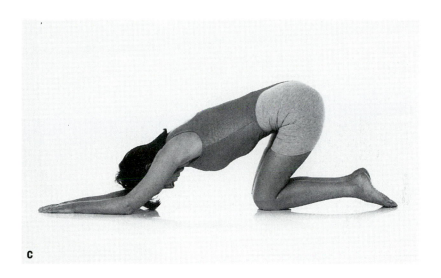

c

4. *Stretch out (c).*

Exercises for your inner thighs

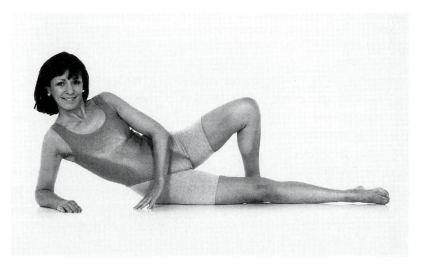

1. *Lie on one side, as shown.*

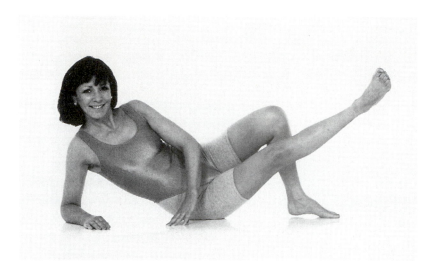

2. *Keeping your legs closely together, raise the front leg and lower eight times.*
3. *Rest for a few seconds. Repeat the exercise sixteen times.*
4. *Change sides.*
5. *Stretch out by putting the soles of your feet together, sit tall and press your thighs out towards the floor.*

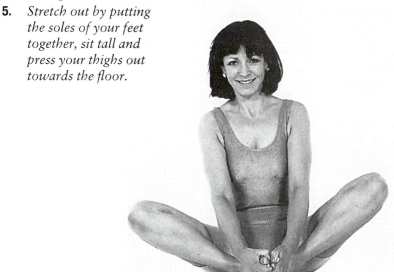

• • • • • • • • • • • • • •

Exercises for your stomach

The basic crunch

This is your basic stomach exercise. If you are new to it, only do two sets of basic crunch, rest, and stretch out. (A set is eight crunch movements.) If you are used to exercise, do two sets and repeat three times, resting and stretching in between.

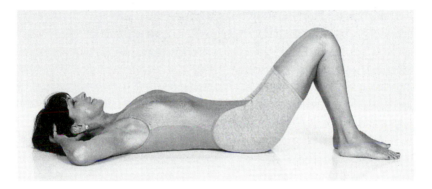

1. *It is important that you protect your back through all these exercises. You should feel the small of your back on the floor. Do not think in terms of lifting your head, think instead of* pressing *your abdomen down through your spine to the floor.*

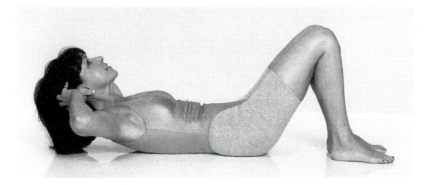

2. *Support your head with one hand, reach out with the other towards your knee or thigh. DO THIS SLOWLY. Do eight or sixteen, depending on your fitness, rest and repeat changing hands.*

• • • • • • • • • • • • • •

The crossover crunch

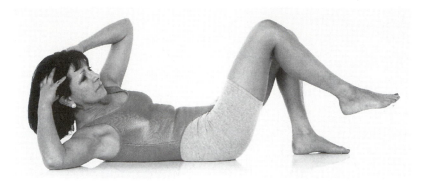

1. *Lie with your head supported by both hands, leaving your neck free of tension. To test that you are not straining your neck, you should be able to count to ten while performing this exercise.*
2. *Inhale before you start. Exhale, and lift your upper body AT THE SAME TIME as you lift your right foot off the floor SIX INCHES. Slightly angle your opposite shoulder towards the right knee. Do six and change sides.*

NOTE: *If you lift your leg any higher into your chest, you will be using your thigh muscles to help you, so resist. By lifting just a few inches, you will keep all the effort in your stomach muscles.*

3. *Rest, then repeat sixteen times each side.*

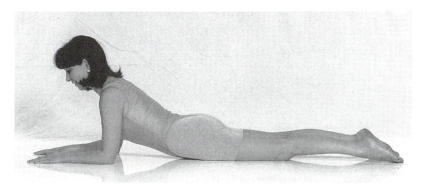

4. *Turn over to stretch out.*

• • • • • • • • • • • • •

The quarter sit-up

This is a far more advanced exercise. If you prefer, rest your legs on a chair.

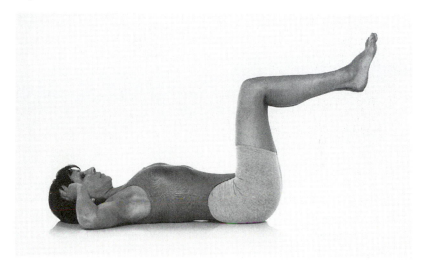

1. *Take starting position as above.*

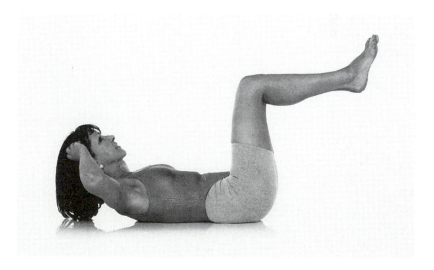

2. *Breathe in, then as you breathe out lift yourself up, including your shoulderblades, and lower again. The idea is to keep your*

• • • • • • • • • • • • •

legs steady and not let your knees roll in towards your chest, and to press your stomach downwards. You should try not to tug on your head or neck. Do eight or sixteen, rest and repeat.

If you feel that you could do more exercise, go through the entire sequence of exercises one more time. BRILLIANT!

Recording Your Progress

As you go through the fortnight, keeping a personal record of your weight and measurements is an excellent way of seeing how you are progressing. You will want not only to weigh yourself, but keep track of your measurements too. Knowing what you weigh alone is no real indicator of whether you have a good figure.

Measuring yourself is almost as much of a challenge as weighing yourself, but it's necessary in order to seee where weight has been lost from (if indeed you lose any weight, as the exercise plan should ensure you tone up and lose inches, even if not weight), and what areas to focus on. Weight loss can be depressing if you've kept to your diet for weeks, you know that the pounds are disappearing, yet your body has all the same bulges.

How to measure yourself

While you still want to weigh yourself too, get out that tape measure and have a good measuring session, concentrating on the following points around your body:

upper arms _____

upper chest (armpits) _____

bust _____

under bust _____

waist _____

navel _____

pubic bone _____

hips _____

upper thigh _____

above knee _____

calf _____

ankle _____

• • • • • • • • • • • • • •

Fill in this week's measurements, followed by next week's for comparison.

RECORD OF PROGRESS

WEEK ONE			WEEK TWO
Date		. . . .	. . . .
Weight		. . . . st/kg . . . . lb/g	. . . . st/kg . . . . lb/g
Upper arm	(left)	. . . . in/cm	. . . . in/cm
	(right)	. . . . in/cm	. . . . in/cm
Upper chest		. . . . in/cm	. . . . in/cm
Bust		. . . . in/cm	. . . . in/cm
Under bust		. . . . in/cm	. . . . in/cm
Waist		. . . . in/cm	. . . . in/cm
Navel		. . . . in/cm	. . . . in/cm
Pubic bone		. . . . in/cm	. . . . in/cm
Hips		. . . . in/cm	. . . . in/cm
Upper thigh	(left)	. . . . in/cm	. . . . in/cm
	(right)	. . . . in/cm	. . . . in/cm
Above knee	(left)	. . . . in/cm	. . . . in/cm
	(right)	. . . . in/cm	. . . . in/cm
Calf	(left)	. . . . in/cm	. . . . in/cm
	(right)	. . . . in/cm	. . . . in/cm
Ankle	(left)	. . . . in/cm	. . . . in/cm
	(right)	. . . . in/cm	. . . . in/cm

NOTE: *You may find that in the second week your bust measurement appears smaller. This is more likely to mean that you have lost fat from your back rather than that your breasts themselves have got smaller! This is why I recommend that you also measure above and below your bust for comparison.*

• • • • • • • • • • • •

Getting Started

Take an honest look at yourself

Most of us are pretty negative about our looks. We insist that there's nothing we're happy with, but is that really true? Let's start with your weight.

Stand in front of a full-length mirror wearing underwear and a well-fitting T-shirt or vest. We're going to judge your weight first from how you look. You might feel heavy, but where does the weight settle? Everyone knows her own body from how her clothes fit, but it never ceases to amaze me that people still judge their figures by what the scales say. *You must forget this!* Your weight doesn't tell you what you look like.

Hold a hand-mirror and take a look at your back view. Does your bottom really need to be smaller, or is it simply lacking tone?

Your back

I suggested wearing a close-fitting T-shirt or vest because it shows up the state of your back. Many women put on weight from the top down, and fat is often stored on the upper back and under the arms. We all have sheets of powerful muscles which allow us to do a whole range of arm movements, but when these muscles get slack they can also manifest themselves as a flabby back which causes unsightly bulges.

Bras highlight the problem because their very nature means that they have to fit closely. If you have a lot of over- and underhang, don't wear tight tops.

Your front

The same goes for your front view. If your top is going to be revealing, you need a smooth line underneath, so no lace or bows on your bra. Choose one which encases your whole breast, and definitely don't wear balcony or uplift bras under bodies or T-shirts. They emphasize any spare breast flesh which might not be in the first flush of youth!

The only people who have genuinely pert, uplifted breasts are about fifteen. Due to the predominance of TV pro- grammes portraying beachloads of silky siliconed beauties, and the fact that breasts are always covered up, lifted up or squeezed into shapes Mother Nature never intended, we should be forgiven for thinking we're falling short if ours are droopy (or 'soft', as a high-class corsetière put it rather delicately), small or mismatching. Your bosom is there, so you might as well make the most of it, and a good bustline is a sign of youthfulness.

If you're small, don't make the mistake of thinking that you don't need support. Always wear a good bra.

Keep reappraising the situation

It's extraordinary that some women buy the same bra size for as long as forty years. Even if your weight has not fluctuated, there's a huge difference between the ages of twenty-five and forty-five in breast terms, and even if your measurement is the same, the way your flesh has settled could be very different. Remember that the measurement round your bust takes in a lot more than just breast tissue. It includes your back and underarms, so check every two or three years that your cup size hasn't altered. *Having a well- fitted bra makes a world of difference to your outline and figure.*

• • • • • • • • • • • • • •

Your stomach

In my last book, *5 Days to a Flatter Stomach*, I talked about causes of a big stomach other than fat. Do read it and follow the suggestions if you suffer from a big stomach and aren't overweight.

Holding ourselves in goes without saying. I think we start to learn how to do this about the age of fourteen, and keep doing it. What a pain. And you can always be sure that the minute you forget yourself and let everything go for a second, all your friends suddenly appear! But what if, despite your valiant efforts, you either get your period or eat something which bloats you out just when you want to look good?

BUY A GIRDLE

It isn't an admission of defeat, and indeed it's a sensible way to give back your confidence and a smooth line under that skirt you've been aching to wear. Buy either a light-control pantie girdle or something a little more heavy-duty, but buy a good one! Don't wait until you need it and the shops are shut.

Your legs

Good legs are classy and an essential part of looking fabulous. What are yours like?

During the past fifteen years or so, there's been a vague feeling of 'Political incorrectness' in the suggestion that men like to look at a pretty leg in a flattering shoe. 'Grunge' fashions, clumpy boots and long skirts have all contributed to women losing interest in their lower legs, though for some reason the spotlight has swung upwards to our thighs. Today's exercise excesses have developed muscular calves and thick ankles, not to mention large thighs, and I think it's a shame that so little interest is shown in the part of the legs everyone sees.

If you have problem legs, or even if you don't, here is what you must do:

• • • • • • • • • • • • • •

1. Follow the foot and leg exercises given on page 56, every day.
2. Keep your legs permanently hair-free and moisturized.
3. Keep your feet immaculate – it will give you a psychological boost.
4. Reduce puffy ankles by drinking two extra pints of water a day – strange though it may seem, water helps reduce fluid retention.
5. Wear dark-coloured tights, and wear tights and shoes of the same colour – this makes your legs look longer and slimmer.

Your feet

Feet can be a sadly neglected area, but not something you can afford to miss. In a crowded life, it's enough that we have to be faced with even the simplest daily beauty routine, never mind adding our hands and feet to the list! It's all too easy to shove on a pair of shoes and it's a case of 'out of sight and out of mind'.

However, rather like the old chestnut about wearing clean knickers in case you have an accident, neglecting your feet in the hope that nobody will ever see them is fraught with hazards. I once worked with a glamorous and immaculate woman, known and admired for her designer suits, expensive haircuts and lacquered nails. One hot summer's afternoon she arrived for a meeting in the usual eye-catching ensemble, but unfortunately, she was also wearing open-toed sandals and had bare legs. At one stage in the proceedings I looked down at the floor and was alarmed to see a set of gnarled, yellow toes poking out from her shoes, and two appallingly dry and cracked heels. I simply couldn't believe my eyes, and neither could anyone else once I'd drawn their attention to it! This wasn't just an oversight, it was long-term, serious neglect, and what's more it marked her out for ever with her gleeful colleagues as a person who was all 'top show'. It was years ago, but whenever we get together and her name comes up, all we can remember about her is her dreadful feet!

Don't get caught out. A weekly pedicure should take no more than twenty minutes.

Your hands and nails

It's no good having long, strong nails if they look like something you'd find on the end of a parrot's claws. Long nails are fine if they look as if you have deliberately cultivated them that way. They're not fine if they look as if they're only long because you can't get round to cutting them. Ragged and dry cuticles are also signs of neglect, and the Fabulous Woman doesn't neglect *anything*.

On the other hand, short nails can be either a disaster or chic, depending on the state of them. If they look short because you like them that way, you take care of them and they shine healthily, that's great. If they are short because you've either bitten them down to the quick or been laying the patio with your bare hands, not so great. At the end of the day, long or short, it doesn't matter as long as your hands look cared about.

During this plan, you will be doing a proper home manicure and giving yourself daily nourishing treatments, so if your hands are a disaster, take heart. Whatever they look like now, they will be looking *better*.

Your face

Your face gets some pretty rough treatment, and it gets all the criticism as well. You can't change what you've got in the next fortnight, but you can make a huge difference to the way you look.

- Do your eyebrows need plucking?
- Does your upper lip need waxing or depilation?
- Have you many spots?
- Is your complexion dull and lifeless?
- Is your skin grimy? (Test with cotton-wool soaked in a skin freshener.)
- Does your make-up need an overhaul?

During the next two weeks we will tackle your face together. You will have a combination of exfoliation, masks, hair-removal sessions and deep-cleanse and moisturizing treatments. An evening is set aside for you to try out new make-up techniques, although I never hold with trying a totally new look for an important event.

By combining these methods with a good diet and plenty of exercise, I can guarantee that you will look and feel like a whole new person in a fortnight's time.

Your neck

It's extraordinary how a woman's neck can let her down. We pay attention to our faces and hair and the neck somehow gets forgotten.

If you're young, and by that I mean anything from sixteen to about twenty, I urge you with all my heart to start to care for your neck. By the time you're thirty or forty, if your neck's gone you can't do a thing about it. What do I mean by 'gone'?

Rings round the neck, slack skin which resembles a turkey's, lots of spots and freckles. I know it's not too palatable to talk about it, but this is what anyone's neck ends up like when a) they've spent a life sunbathing; b) they haven't moisturized their neck; and c) they haven't kept their neck clean.

The same applies to your upper chest and shoulders. The area above your bustline gets exposure when you wear low-cut dresses and tops, swimsuits, T-shirts and so on. Start when you're a teenager: put on a nightly covering of a good moisturizer, and *clean it off in the morning*. In fact, keep your neck and chest as scrupulously clean as you would your face.

If you have neglected your neck, don't worry. We all have something we're a bit sensitive about, and all you can do is make sure you minimize further damage by starting to cleanse and moisturize.

Your hair

The Fabulous Woman's hair always looks just right. It doesn't matter if you've been struggling through a gale-force wind or caught in a shower, once you've got the right style

• • • • • • • • • • • • • •

and condition, you can take such minor disasters in your stride.

The basis of lovely hair is a good cut. Does yours need a trim? Split ends and straggly long hair are instant signs of hair which has been forgotten about, and that says a lot about you. Although you're doing most things yourself in the next fortnight, you need a professional cut, so make an appointment now.

However, a complete re-style or major cut is not a good idea right now, unless you are positive that it will make you feel better, or if you have had the style before and want to go back to it. If you are getting ready for a major event it could be disastrous, as you might not be able to think of anything else. Remember too that a completely different hairstyle will throw your clothes choices out of balance, and you have the shape of your face to consider. Unless you really want to go out and buy a lot of new clothes, stick with what you've got until a time when the stakes aren't so high.

For the next fortnight you'll be getting your hair into peak condition with three deep-conditioning sessions, and you can experiment with new products and hair accessories for added glamour.

Don't forget to make appointments for the hairdresser now. You don't want to leave it too late and find you can't get in.

Making a shopping list

You don't want to be making six trips to the chemist because you haven't got something you need. Here is a list of essentials for your home beauty care:

- good cleansing cream or lotion
- tissues
- cotton-wool pads

• • • • • • • • • • • • •

- cotton-buds
- toning lotion or astringent for oily skin
- good daytime moisturizer
- rich night cream
- small bottle of almond oil
- cuticle remover
- hand cream
- exfoliating cream or gel
- rich body moisturizing lotion
- emery boards
- shampoo and conditioner
- hot-oil hair conditioner
- shower hat, bands and clips for your hair
- face mask (I will be giving you ideas for making your own)
- rough skin remover (for feet)
- sisal mitt

This sounds like a lot, but you may have many of these items already. Remember, too, that by doing your own pedicure, manicure and facial, you are saving in the region of £40–£60!

If there is anything else you have discovered about yourself, which you want to see to, make a note of it, and allocate an hour to dealing with it. For example, bikini-line waxing or electrolysis for stubborn facial hair. *Make appointments now!*

Your Beauty Schedule

Any bride will know all about this. Never leave anything chancy to the last minute, because if you make a mistake there's no time to put it right. For example, a friend of mine went for a different hair colour two days before a major selection panel interview for a job of a lifetime, and she was horrified by the result. Needless to say, the hairdresser couldn't fit her in the following day, she tried to put it right herself, failed dismally and went to her interview feeling self-conscious, lacking in confidence and hideous. She wasn't herself, and didn't get the job.

There can be a whole host of minor disasters which none of us ever think about, but which call for a belt-and-braces approach. I never leave anything to the last minute since the time I went to bed exhausted after a gruelling fitness session, too tired to shower off the sweat from my body and my hair, which had gone into corkscrews. The next day I had an important lunch date, but I reckoned that with an early alarm call I'd be up and away, fresh and fragrant in good time.

Imagine my horror to discover a power cut! No hot water, no hairdryer. No good going to a neighbour because the whole district was off for three hours, as it turned out. I washed in cold water and my hair had to hang. Never again. It might sound like a once-in-a-million scenario, but once bitten, twice shy. These days I prepare while the going's good, and repeat it the following day if necessary.

Leaving everything to the last minute is not the Fabulous Woman's style. *You should look and feel perfection itself by the day before, then any final touches you can give your hair and face are a bonus.*

These treatments should be done EVERY DAY:
- Moisturize your body with scented cream (after your bath).
- Thoroughly cleanse, tone and moisturize your face.
- Massage your hands and nails for two minutes with good hand and nail cream.
- Shave your legs.
- Pluck stray hairs from your eyebrows.
- Apply rich body lotion to your shoulders, neck and chest before bed.

These treatments should be done three times a week:
- Gently exfoliate your face.
- Remove hard skin from your feet and massage.
- Soak your nails in hot oil for ten minutes.

These treatments should be done ONCE A WEEK:
- Complete body exfoliation or scrub down.
- Full facial with mask (a mask can be applied twice a week if you have the time).
- Full pedicure.
- Full manicure.
- Hair conditioning, using hot-oil or deep-conditioning treatment which should be left on for a minimum of ten minutes.

As an optional extra, application of fake tan needs to be done about twice a week, depending on the strength of the product you are using.

Working out your timetable

In this book I have set out a timetable which covers everything in one week. It's a good idea to set aside at least half an hour a day for your beauty routine in future; in practice you'll find that you need much less time as you get more experienced at doing everything yourself.

Good grooming doesn't take long. It only takes a long time the first time if you've let everything go, and who doesn't from time to time? A personal crisis, a bereavement, illness, staying away from home where you don't have your own things to hand . . . these all contribute to the slow neglect which eventually gets us down.

Stop the rot. Use the ideas in this book to get yourself back in control, and after that it's simple maintenance.

If you're not planning a special date, it's nice to set aside an evening for playing with make-up. Even if you're not the type to wear much, it's important to know how to emphasize your good features and cover any blemishes you might have, so don't ignore the make-up section completely.

Look after your skin. Treat it well and it will pay you back richly in terms of compliments and reputation.

• • • • • • • • • • • • • • •

Day One

Start today as you will every day on this plan, with a good wake-up stretch by an open window.

1. *Inhale through your nose to a count of four as you raise your arms above your head. Clasp your hands and press upwards. Breathe out to a further count of four as you lower your arms.*

2. *Clasp your hands behind your back. Drop your head and pull your arms downwards, feeling the stretch in your neck and shoulders. Hold for ten seconds.*

3. *Clasp your hands in front of you, round your chest and drop your head. Press away from you, feeling as if someone has hold of your hands and is gently pulling away. Bend your knees slightly and tuck your bottom under. Hold for ten seconds.*

4. *Repeat the first stretch.*

Your morning beauty routine

Every day you will be tackling some beauty task, but in the morning rush you must never forget that your face and neck need attention. After a night's sleep, your skin had shed its dead cells, and they will need to be removed with more than just a splash of water.

Tying your hair back off your face, apply cleansing lotion (or wash-off cleanser if your prefer the feel of water) and cleanse twice. Apply toning lotion, to remove all traces of cleansing cream, and check that the cotton wool is quite clear of any grime. Apply a thin film of daytime moisturizer.

Your exercises today

Start with a brisk walk if possible. Your exercises are on page 54. Try to do the whole sequence before you have your shower or breakfast; it should take no more than fifteen minutes.

Your beauty routine tonight

I always love the part of the week when I lock the bathroom door, put on some music and set about giving myself a good scrub down!

It sounds terrible, doesn't it? As if we spend all week getting more and more grubby and this is our first clean-up, but we all know it's not like that. Modern-day pollution means that few of us can keep our skins clean for long, and our beauty suffers as a result. Listen to what our beauty expert Amanda Fredericks had to say:

'I see women pretty well as Nature intended. They strip off for massages and facials, and I've stopped being amazed at how badly some people look after themselves. Some clients, for instance, are wealthy women who pride themselves on their appearance and designer clothes, but you'd be amazed at the number who have really dirty ears!

'Another thing I see is dirty necks, full of blackheads. The client looks fine, but when she leans back and her neck is extended, the creases of her neck are sometimes actually grimy. People's backs can be dreadful, in the bit they can't reach. I think it's all down to showers. People stand in them and the water just runs down and doesn't go under their boobs or necks. A good steam session and exfoliating once a week is all people need.'

• • • • • • • • • • • • • •

Cleanse and tone

You will need:

- band and grips for hair
- eye make-up remover
- cotton-wool pads
- cleansing cream
- toning lotion
- wash-off exfoliating grains or cream for face
- rich night moisturizer

1. Tie your hair back from your face and secure with a hair band or grips.
2. Using your eye make-up remover and a cotton-wool pad, gently take off your eye make-up using a downward sweep. Do not drag the skin around the eyes or lids. Repeat until there is not a trace of colour or masacara left.
3. Take a good dollop of cleansing cream and smooth all over face and neck. Massage in, using an upward circular movement with both hands.
4. Using a large cotton-wool pad which has been held under the cold tap or with a splash of toning lotion on it, remove the cleanser using an upward sweeping movement. *Never take make-up off downwards*.
5. Repeat the procedure. Your skin should now be clean, but repeat once more if necessary.
6. Put some toning lotion on a cotton-wool pad. Sweep it over your face in an upward movement, removing all traces of cleanser. Go right up to the hairline.
7. Dampen your face by splashing with warm (not hot) water. Take a palmful of exfoliating grains or cream and gently rub into your skin, taking care to avoid the eye area. Massage gently for one minute. Rinse off with warm water.
8. Splash with cold water and pat dry.
9. Place a dollop of night moisturizer or lotion in one palm and smooth it between your hands. Do not apply directly to the skin or rub in. Smooth both hands over your face without dragging. Pat with fingertips.

BEAUTY THERAPIST'S TIP: *'Never leave your make-up on for more than twelve hours. Try to have at least one make-up-free day every week, but still cleanse, tone and moisturize to remove dirt and grime.'*

Body exfoliation
METHOD 1
You will need:

- hair band or grips
- a tube or tub of a good exfoliating body cream, lotion or grains
- depilatory cream or lady's razor (for hair removal on legs and underarms)
- Massage oil and rich body cream (see page 88)

1. Tie your hair back and secure with a band or grips, or use a bath hat.
2. Standing naked on a towel, take a good palmful of your exfoliating cream or grains into slightly wet hands.
3. Starting at one foot and using both hands, lift foot onto a higher surface (to save your back!) and start to rub the cream or grains into your foot. Use circular movements from back to front, the hands working together. Work up the leg and rub as briskly as you can.
4. Take another palmful of exfoliating cream or grains into damp hands. Don't forget the backs of your thighs (important for cellulite), and your bottom. You should be massaging really briskly and with a good pressure by now, and even feel that you are a little breathless with the effort.
5. Take another palmful. Carry on up the body, not forgetting under your bust and your stomach.
6. Take another palmful. Wet your body slightly if this procedure feels at all dry, as it all depends on the type of exfoliating preparation you are using. Now do your arms, and the backs of your shoulders. Keep massaging as hard as you can. Do your neck, back and front, right up to your hairline. Don't worry, it's all going to be rinsed off in a moment and your skin will feel like silk!

This whole procedure should take between five and ten minutes, which is a guide to how long you should stay in

• • • • • • • • • • • • • •

each area. Go back over your whole body and give one last hard scrub.

METHOD 2
You will need:
- sisal mitt (available from chemists)
- good quality soap
- massage oil and rich body cream (see page 88)

This is the method I prefer, as I started treating myself to a sisal mitt scrub long before exfoliating grains were heard of. You can do this in a shower or bath using a sisal mitt which is sold in chemists for under £2.

1   Rub the bar of soap on to the sisal mitt first. Apply to your limbs, starting with your feet, and scrub in a circular motion with one hand. You will get beautifully soapy, and when you wash or shower the lather away, your skin will feel like silk.
2   Stand in a nice hot shower and rinse thoroughly.
3   Now I suggest you lie in a scented bath for about ten minutes.

Getting rid of the hair on your legs and underarms
I recently asked a group of women what annoyed them most about their bodies, apart from the shape, and they all agreed that it was knowing that they were hairy! Having a good go at leg hair, eyebrows and underarm hair made everyone feel much lighter. After tonight's treatment you'll start tomorrow feeling fresher.

It's sometimes said that you shouldn't shave your legs, but I have never had a problem with it. Waxing your legs means you have to wait for the hair to grow to a certain length, and frankly, I don't want to see a hair on my legs – ever! I run a razor over my legs every day when I shower, it takes about ten seconds for each leg and they are permanently smooth and hair-free. I suggest you give it a go.

• • • • • • • • • • • • •

1. Make sure your razor is new and sharp.
2. Using either soap or shaving cream, lather the entire leg.
3. Using a long stroke, start at your ankle and do one stroke to the knee.
4. Rinse the razor between strokes.
5. Carry on with the lower leg, shave above the knee and thigh if you are including this area, then repeat on the opposite leg. Rinse in cool, clear water (preferably under the shower).
6. Repeat the procedure on your underarm area.

Always use an unperfumed or lightly perfumed body lotion over the legs after shaving, and do not use deodorant under the armpits immediately afterwards.

Alternatively, use a depilatory cream. These are not as fashionable as they once were, but the beauty of them is that you simply apply the cream, put the kettle on or do something else, and then rinse the cream off and the hair's gone. They tend to smell a bit, but it doesn't last long.

Applying massage oil and body lotion
When you get out of your bath, make sure you shower yourself down with clean water, or use a jug with fresh water from the tap. You don't want a soapy or greasy residue on your skin.

Mix a little of the body lotion with a teaspoonful of almond oil for a very rich lotion, and massage in well, rather as you did for the exfoliating. If you don't like the greasiness, omit the oil. Try to spend a little time without your clothes, to allow the lotion to take maximum effect.

Talcum powder can be applied to all the creases, such as under your bust and at the tops of your legs, but be sparing. Talc which is applied too thickly can go into lumps, which are then highly irritating for your skin.

Your neck, shoulders and decolleté
If you sleep alone, it is a good idea to massage some rich body lotion or oil into your neck, shoulders and chest area.

• • • • • • • • • • • • •

Otherwise I suggest you perform this massage an hour or so before bed, relax somewhere warm where you can leave off your dressing-gown, and then remove the excess before you go to bed.

Your nails
You will be doing a full manicure tomorrow, but for now you need to get into the habit of a good hand and nail massage.

Your skin will be warm from the bath, so as soon as you have finished moisturizing your body, take a little body lotion, add some oil, and rub it between your hands. Massage each finger and nail, paying particular attention to the nail bed, which is where the growth of each nail begins. It isn't much use nourishing the nail itself, which is dead, but by promoting growth at the base you will notice the benefits in the weeks to come.

Try to get into the habit of a few minutes' nail massage every day, and keep a small tube of either hand cream or specialist cuticle nourishing cream in your handbag, and if you find yourself waiting somewhere, do a couple of minutes of nail massage.

Good! You have reached the end of your first day of the Fabulous in a Fortnight plan and you should be feeling better already. Have your supper and get a good night's sleep.

Checklist
1. You should have everything you will need in the way of beauty items together now, for the next fortnight.

    Even if you have done this already, check the shade of lipstick you are thinking of wearing. I once had a lovely white dress with a strip of pink around the shoulders; it wasn't until the day I first wore it that I realized how badly my own rather bluey-pink lipsticks clashed with the orangey-pink of the border, which being close to my face made the problem even more obvious. Even experienced clothes horses get caught out on this one, so don't leave this detail to the last minute.

• • • • • • • • • • • • • •

2. THINK OF EVERYTHING AND PLAN AHEAD. While I'll deal with this in more detail later on, if you are working towards an occasion which means a lot to you, check for instance that you can handle all the bits and pieces you'll be carrying. For example, you might find yourself at an outdoors event on a windy day, and be caught having to use one hand to hold on to your hat, leaving just the other for your handbag, glass and to manage your hemline! A good rehearsal is never wasted.

Your Meals for Day One

BREAKFAST
2 slices wholemeal toast
1 teaspoon marmalade or jam
butter from allowance (*Cut a block of butter into 7 g/¹/₄ oz pats and use one a day on your morning or evening toast – see page 31*)

MID-MORNING
150 ml/5 fl oz skimmed milk *or*
decaffeinated coffee made with 100 ml/3½ fl oz skimmed milk *or*
Banana milkshake: 100 ml/3½ fl oz skimmed milk and 1 banana, blended together

MAIN MEAL
Mushroom Medley Risotto (page 187) *or*
roast or grilled chicken breast with potatoes, carrots, broccoli

Poached Stuffed Peach (page 214)
tea or coffee

LIGHT MEAL
1 jacket potato
25 g/1 oz grated cheese
salad from salads selection (pages 199–211)

SUPPER
2 slices wholemeal toast
1 teaspoon jam or Marmite
bedtime drink
mineral water

• • • • • • • • • • • • • •

Day Two

Start the day as you did yesterday, with your full wake-up stretch. Remember to breathe correctly, in through your nose and out through your mouth. Your breathing has been shallow while you were asleep, so now's the time to stand by the window and really fill those lungs with good, fresh air and oxygen. Enjoy it, it will wake you up.

Don't forget your proper cleanse, tone and moisturize routine. It really pays to keep working at your skin condition.

Your exercises today

Have you promised yourself any exercise before breakfast? Even if it's wet outdoors, or chilly or windy, wrap up against it and get out. Don't let anything stand in your way. There are worse things than being a little damp, and you must tell yourself that it's worth it. Every moment you are walking, you are boosting your metabolic rate and using up those calories. At least get a twenty minute brisk walk.

If you can't leave the house, change into something loose and comfortable ready for your floor exercises.

Your beauty routine tonight
Beautiful nails
I always believe in killing two birds with one stone. Doing a thorough manicure will take you about twenty minutes to

half an hour, depending on whether you choose to add nail polish, so use the time to condition your hair.

Using one of the hot-oil conditioning treatments you bought, follow the instructions for preparation of your hair. Remember to get out of your clothes and into a bath robe or dressing-gown first. Apply the conditioner to your damp hair and wrap with cling film.

Most of us aspire to elegant, perfectly manicured hands with long nails. Unfortunately, not many people have them, and the unfairness of it all seems to be that the girls who look after their nails the least seem to always have ten perfect talons while you sit fiddling and filing and soaking your nails half the day and end up with a set of pathetically brittle, broken or flaky efforts, all different lengths. So what's going wrong?

There is no magic formula for beautiful nails. However, there is a lot you can do to maintain and improve them, and you have to start with nails which look healthy and cared for.

Just because someone's nails are long doesn't necessarily mean that they are attractive. If they are long because you can't be bothered to file them, it will show. If your nails are short because they are either bitten or used to hard wear and tear, it will also show. Short nails need to look as if they were intended that way, or they will say a lot about you which you might not be pleased about.

On average, nails grow at about 4mm a month. Of course, nail growth varies from person to person – it is greater in spring and summer and in young people. It is also stimulated in pregnancy when hormones are running riot, and many pregnant women suddenly find their nails, skin and hair in the best condition ever.

If your nails are a disgrace, or you think they are, you can make a huge difference to them in a fortnight. Despite the fact that you can't hope for much nail growth in two weeks, by simply dealing with excess cuticle, and treating the area around the nail bed, you will expose more of the nail and make it appear much longer.

• • • • • • • • • • • • • •

If your nails are already long and lovely, this treatment still needs to be done to keep them that way, especially a nightly nail soak.

You will need:

- emery board
- cuticle cream
- bowl of warm soapy water
- hoof stick or orange stick
- cuticle clippers
- towel and tissues

It is better to file your nails than to cut them. Steel files are best left for toenails, as they can break or flake your fingernails.

Always file your nails from the outside edge to the middle, trying to achieve a nice smooth curve. Never file back and forth, as this can cause the nail layers to split.

Most importantly, your nails should be the same length. Don't hang on to one nice long nail in the hope that the others will catch up – they won't!

1. File each nail from the side to the centre, holding the emery board at an angle of 45 degrees.
2. Holding the file vertically, file the top of the nail in a downward movement, using a gentle 'brushing' action.
3. Apply a small amount of cuticle cream to each cuticle. Massage in with circular movements of the thumb.
4. Soak fingertips in a bowl of warm, soapy water. Leave each hand for about five minutes, then remove and dry thoroughly. (Alternatively, this can be done in a hot bath.)
5. Push back the cuticles very gently with a hoof stick or orange stick. Trim any excess cuticle or hangnail carefully with cuticle clippers. (*Some beauticians say you should never cut the cuticle. In this procedure you are trimming away excess dead skin and not harming the cuticle itself. Take care not to dig too deeply, or you might damage the nail bed and leave the cuticle raw.*)

• • • • • • • • • • • • •

6. **NAIL SOAK**

   Using a small pot which can withstand heat, fill with either a little olive oil or almond oil. Microwave for 1 minute or stand in a dish of boiling water (I stand mine on the wood-burning stove – it gets hot in about two minutes).

   Soak each set of nails while you do something else, like reading the paper, watching television or eating with the other hand! Blot your nails to remove excess, but leave enough oil for a massage. Repeat with the other hand.

7. Blot both hands and start to massage. Follow the procedure as for last night, spending a good minute on each hand. Try not to wash off the oil for an hour or so.

   If you have to do some jobs round the house now, I suggest you wear some disposable gloves. These are inexpensive and I find them indispensable for all kinds of fiddly jobs, from arranging flowers to polishing the furniture, if I want to stop things getting covered with oily fingermarks.

BUFFING

Healthy, shiny nails are the best finishing touch for a healthy, natural look. They will enhance every outfit, from a cocktail dress to a sweater and shorts.

Buffing doesn't dry out your nails and is an excellent way of stimulating the circulation and smoothing the nail surface. If your nails are in poor condition, it is far better to treat them to a good buffing than to try to disguise them with polish.

You will need:

- rich hand cream or cuticle cream
- nail buffer
- cuticle oil
- cotton-wool ball
- toning lotion
- clear nail polish

1. Dot each nail with a small amount of hand or cuticle cream.
2. Buff with a firm downward movement, from the base of the nail to the tip. Lift the buffer after each stroke.
3. Spend about half a minute on each nail. Keep the movements short and firm rather than using a scrubbing action.

• • • • • • • • • • • • • • •

4. Apply cuticle oil round each cuticle and massage in with the ball of your thumb.
5. Using the cotton-wool ball with a touch of toning lotion wipe the nail dry – the cuticle retains the oil.
6. Apply clear liquid nail polish.

APPLYING POLISH

Are you one of those women who believe that air vents in cars were put there to dry your nail polish? Have you ever sat in your car, engine running and stomach churning, applying nail polish with shaky hands?

Always do your nail polish a couple of days beforehand, or whenever you've plenty of time to relax and get it perfect. If you then have to repeat the procedure or touch up any chips, you won't need more than a couple of minutes. It's better to leave your nails bare than to apply nail polish scrappily.

If you are trying a new outfit or a colour you haven't worn before, I suggest you try your new nail colour now. It's easy to make a mistake, to find that the colour either doesn't really match your dress after all or it's just not you. Remember the whole purpose of the next two weeks is to practise, try out and try on. *Make your mistakes in private!*

1. Follow the instructions for nail buffing.
2. Using your coloured polish, apply it in three strokes, starting with a central downward stroke.
3. Follow with a stroke either side.
4. If the polish smudges, use an orange stick dipped in some nail polish remover and carefully wipe away.
5. Repeat the coat after the first one has had time to dry.
6. Finish with a top coat which acts as a sealer and protector.

    Ideally, you should leave your nails to dry for about half an hour, or use one of the fast-drying spray products, which speeds up the process.

How can I make a manicure last?

Take each coat of polish under the nail and along the edge of the nail tip. This seals it and prevents water getting in. Every two days add a further top coat, until the coloured nail polish needs redoing completely.

• • • • • • • • • • • •

How can I stop my nails flaking and splitting?
Use treatment products for dryness and use them all the
time. Massage with cuticle cream while you wait for the bus,
watch TV or have your lunch in the office. Never peel off
flaking nails – rub with a dry flannel if they are catching on
your tights, otherwise leave them alone. Massage helps,
although it takes about four months to work. Simply keep
at it – your nails will get better with persistence!

Removing your hair conditioner
When your nails are dry, remove the cling film and thoroughly shampoo your hair several times to remove the
hot-oil conditioning treatment. Dry and style in your usual
way.

If you are not used to conditioning treatments for your
hair – as opposed to applying a normal after-shampoo
conditioner – you might find your hair feels slightly limp
and 'greasy' afterwards. You will soon get used to slightly
softer hair, and of course the deep-conditioning treatment
isn't meant to be done more than once a week. Think of it
as a long drink for your thirsty hair.

I'll be talking more about your hair in a couple of days'
time.

Good! You have finished your second day and should be
feeling even better. Are you?

If you are hoping to lose weight by the end of two weeks,
I trust you aren't finding the diet too hard. If you are hungry,
do eat something, as long as it is starchy. Raw vegetables
and fruit are all very well, but they don't satisfy in the long
run. Try half a piece of toast, a banana, half a bowl of cereal
with skimmed milk – or even cold potatoes!

You will be glad when you are slimmer, and proud of
yourself for sticking with it. We all like to tuck in to the odd
piece of cake, but if you've ever been in the position of
starting on a whole cake, or packet of biscuits, knowing you
won't stop until you've finished it, think how you'll feel in
the morning.

• • • • • • • • • • • • • •

Checklist

1. Check tomorrow's meal plans and see if you have everything in.
2. Check tomorrow's beauty treatment, which is a facial, and make sure you have everything you need.
3. Have you done your exercises today? If not, why not? Did you run out of time or motivation? You MUST try to keep to your exercise plan, because it's the only way you'll get the figure you've always dreamed of. I know it's easier to stay in. I know you deserve a break after a dreadful day. Half an hour or an hour of exercise isn't the whole evening wasted, far from it. Make a resolution to do a bit more tomorrow.
4. Do you have anything which needs to go to the cleaner's?
5. If you are wearing something old, which might have been stored or not worn for some months, check for moth damage or repairs which you might have forgotten about. Maybe you had a food stain on the cuff last time you wore it, and forgot to get it seen to before you put it away for the winter? There's nothing worse than finding out the moment you put it on, and desperately running a flannel under the tap to try to scrub it off. It never works. Check now.

Your Meals for Day Two

BREAKFAST
25 g/1 oz unsweetened cereal (Rice Crispies, Special K, cornflakes)
150 ml/5 fl oz skimmed milk
tea or decaffeinated coffee
mineral water

MID-MORNING
1 apple, orange or pear
tea or decaffeinated coffee
mineral water

MAIN MEAL
Macaroni Cheese with Tomatoes (page 185) *or*
Chicken Roulade with Layered Vegetables (page 174)
banana, fromage frais

LIGHT MEAL

1 jacket potato with 100 g/4 oz cottage cheese, colourful mixed
salad with watercress, grated carrot and sweetcorn *or*
Cottage cheese and fruit salad: arrange 1 sliced apple, 12 grapes, 12
orange and grapefruit segments round a plate. Spoon 100 g/4 oz
cottage cheese on to a bed of watercress in the centre. *or*
1 round light cream cheese and grape wholemeal sandwich

mixed fruit salad *or*
3 pieces of fresh fruit

SUPPER

2 slices wholemeal toast
1 teaspoon jam or Marmite
bedtime drink
mineral water

Day Three

How are you feeling this morning? Lighter I hope, and fresher after some decent sleep and beauty treatments.

How is your diet going? Some of the portions can seem small if you're used to hearty eating, but give it another few days and you'll find your stomach's adjusted to it, and you won't feel like such large amounts.

The diet is important because it is devised for energy and beauty. Years ago it was universally accepted that you felt tired, washed out and hungry on a diet. A top professor of dietetics and nutrition who was the guru of the 1960s even wrote that 'carbohydrates should be cut down, and you should eat as much as you like of butter, meat, eggs, fish and cream'. Hardly believable nowadays. Carbohydrates have lost their 'stodgy' label, and are now seen as low-calorie, versatile, convenient and chic. Indeed, with today's interest in exercise, it is vital that you eat more carbohydrate so you can keep going for longer, while reducing your intake of fat and protein.

Another piece of advice from the sixties was to restrict fluid intake to no more than six small cups of tea or coffee a day. This advice was wildly wrong, but the thinking behind it was that fluid adds to your weight. Well, yes. Stand on a pair of scales and slowly drink a pint of water and you'll see the needle rise! You'll have gained weight, but not fat! Fluid is essential for health and beauty, it keeps the skin plumped out and so avoids wrinkles, it helps the stomach digest food and, best of all, it helps guard against bloating. Yes! It seems strange to say that fluid retention is helped by drinking extra water, but it's true.

Remember your wake-up stretch and floor exercises. Even if you don't have time to do the full set, two minutes will be better than nothing.

Your beauty routine tonight

Before you get down to your beauty routine, have you done your exercises tonight? Turn back to this morning's instructions and repeat them. They should take about ten minutes.

> **THE FULL FACIAL**
>
> Tonight you are going to give yourself a full facial, including a herbal steam treatment and a home-made face pack or mask (or use a bought product if you prefer).
>
> Never have a facial directly before a special event o r when it matters to look your best. Deep cleansing can leave your face looking raw for a day, so always allow a day's grace for your skin to settle down.

You will need

- facial mask (or you can make your own, see below)
- cleansing cream
- toning lotion
- exfoliating grains or cream
- handful of dried herbs – sage, basil, mint, thyme (optional)
- cotton wool and tissues
- 'spritzer' water spray (*you can use tap water in a household spray gun if you like*)
- eye pads (*put wet cotton-wool pads in the fridge for half an hour first*)
- rich moisturizing cream or lotion for night use
- eye cream or light daytime moisturizer
- almond oil
- hair bands and grips

YOUR FACE PACK OR MASK

You can easily buy a sachet of facial mask at any chemist's, but you need to know your skin type first. If you want to be sure of not irritating your skin, the best bet is to make your own mask at home, with the sort of ingredients most of us have to hand. Here are just two of my favourites:

Honey and egg mask

You will need 1 egg white, 1 tablespoon clear honey and 50g/2oz rice flour.

1. In a small bowl, lightly beat the egg white. Add the honey and flour and mix to a smooth paste.
2. Apply to clean skin, over the face and neck. It is a good idea to have steamed your face first, so your pores will be open. Leave for ten to fifteen minutes.
3. Wash off with cold water and pat dry.

Banana Mask

You will need 1 ripe banana, 25 g/1 oz fine oatmeal and 1 teaspoon clear honey.

1. Mash the banana in a bowl until soft.
2. Stir in the oatmeal and honey and mix to a paste.
3. Smooth over clean face and neck. Relax for fifteen minutes.
4. Wash off with clean, cold water. Pat dry and apply moisturizer.

The facial procedure is as follows:
1. Prepare your chosen face mask (see above).
2. Tie your hair securely off your face and neck.
3. Thoroughly cleanse your face twice, using damp cotton wool or tissues to remove the cream.
4. Tone.

5. Using your exfoliating grains or cream, thoroughly but gently scrub the face for one minute. Rinse thoroughly in warm water and pat dry.

6. Tone to remove traces of exfoliator.

7. Take a normal-sized mixing bowl. Pour in boiling water to come about halfway up the bowl, adding a good handful of the dried herbs of your choice, if using.

8. Cover your head with a towel and lean over the bowl for about three minutes. This treatment opens your pores to remove any trapped dirt and helps eliminate blackheads.

9. Pat skin dry. Study your face in a magnifying mirror for blackheads, and gently press them out if necessary.

10. Using a little warm almond oil, gently massage your face, avoiding your eye area, for about two minutes. Take care not to drag the skin, or pull it.

11. Using toner, remove the oil.

12. Take the cold eye pads from the fridge and keep handy.

13. Apply the face mask to your skin while still warm. Lie down and relax with the cold eye pads covering your eyes (this will help reduce any puffiness round the eyes). You might like to lie in a bath while your mask is working.

14. Remove all traces of the mask, and rinse thoroughly with cold water. Pat skin dry.

15. Take a small amount of rich moisturizing lotion or night cream into your palms and mix. Apply to your skin with both hands, using a smoothing and patting action. Using your fingertips, pat into your face.

16. It is a good idea to use a separate eye cream for underneath the eyes, otherwise use a lighter daytime moisturizer to eliminate puffiness.

Good! You have now completed a thorough home facial and should be feeling wonderful. Make sure you have a little supper, and get to bed early because you know there is nothing better for feeling fabulous than your beauty sleep!

Checklist

At the end of this, your third day, take stock for a minute. You need to start thinking about what you're going to be wearing tomorrow, and your accessories.

• • • • • • • • • • • • •

1. Check over your clothes. Is there anything you should be washing? Make a note to do it tomorrow.

2. Is there anything you need to buy, such as more hand cream, body lotion, tissues or tweezers? Do you have small sizes of creams to carry in your handbag?

3. Do you have new tights or stockings in the right shade? How about having some spares in case of accidents when you put them on?

4. If you've decided to have some of the beauty treatments, such as waxing, done professionally, have you made your appointments?

5. How do you feel? Should you be doing a bit more exercise? You've read about posture in the 'Your Image' section (see page 15), but have you practised it?

Well done! Remember that you can become whatever you want to become, and it doesn't take much effort to really make something of yourself. All this effort, all the exercise and dieting and new clothes and hair conditioning will be money down the drain if you forget to smile and look bright and cheerful. A miserable face is something we sometimes can't help, but it will let you down. Nobody wants to get stuck with someone who looks like she might be hard work. Think about this for tomorrow.

You *can* look fabulous, you *can* draw admiring glances and have people talking about you if you believe in yourself. It doesn't take money, it takes confidence. Don't get caught out slouching, chewing, or with your stomach hanging slackly. Most important, never be caught out looking sour.

Practise how you look. Stand tall. Smile.

If you have a tape recorder, it isn't a bad idea to record your voice. Most of us have done this at some time in our lives, and I don't know anyone who wasn't horrified. In truth, we don't usually sound as bad as we fear, but if you have a habit of speaking too quickly, too loudly, or cutting off the ends of your words, it doesn't hurt to be aware of it because it can give the wrong impression. You might think that it's too late to do anything about your voice, but a conscious effort to speak a little more slowly, to pitch your voice down a bit or to speak more clearly can be easily learned in a few days. It's a habit. Do listen to yourself speaking, or ask a friend for an honest opinion.

Your Meals for Day Three

REAKFAST
2 slices wholemeal toast
butter from allowance
1 teaspoon marmalade or jam *or*
1 slice wholemeal toast
butter from allowance
1 boiled egg

MID-MORNING
1 banana

MAIN MEAL
grilled plaice
175 g/6 oz boiled potatoes
2 tablespoons carrots
2 tablespoons peas or broccoli *or*
Thai-style Stir-fried Vegetables (page 192)
Baked Apple and Custard (page 213)
mineral water
tea or decaffeinated coffee

LIGHT MEAL
Herby Stuffed Tomatoes (page 195) *or*
Welsh Rarebit with Tomatoes (page 197) *or*
1 round salad wholemeal sandwich

fruit salad
mineral water

SUPPER
2 digestive biscuits
bedtime drink made with water or skimmed milk

• • • • • • • • • • • • • •

Day Four

Morning warm-up stretch
Go through your three-stretch sequence, as you have done every morning.

Beauty routine
Remember to give yourself a good cleanse, tone and nourish, to clean your skin of dead cells and general debris.

The 'power walk'
Today, try to go for a power walk. What is it? It's a form of walking that uses your upper body as well as your legs, and it means you are using a lot more calories and getting a far better workout in terms of cardiovascular fitness and muscular toning. It's a lot of fun, especially if you can get together with a few friends to keep you company. You need to be somewhere out of the public gaze, unless of course you're an exhibitionist who couldn't give a hoot about what people are thinking!

1. Start off with five minutes of normal walking. Stop for a moment and stretch out your muscles (page 56).
2. Set off again and gather pace. Try to get into a steady rhythm of strides, and bring in your breathing so that you breathe in to four strides and out to six. As you get more puffed you might want to reduce this to in for two counts and out for four. See how you go.
3. Now add arm movements, something like these:

- Sixteen bicep curls (elbow bends). Go 'up–down', one to each strike of the foot.
- Pectoral presses. With elbows at shoulder height, bring hands and elbows to touch and take out again. One movement to each foot strike. Do sixteen.
- Chest presses. Start with hands at shoulder level, reach for the sky and bring down again. Do sixteen.
- Lateral raises. Start with arms hanging down. Raise elbows to the side and lower. Do sixteen.

Drop your arms and keep walking for a minute to rest. Start again, and do the complete sequence of movements, sixteen bicep curls, sixteen pectoral presses, sixteen chest presses and sixteen lateral raises. It is quite tiring, but very good for you, and you're getting slimmer and fitter all the time. Keep resting and repeating, and keep up your walk for at least twenty minutes.

You will find power walking most exhilarating, and I do urge you to try it out today. If it's raining or otherwise inclement, skip on to tonight's exercises and do those instead. Save the power walk for another day!

You mustn't ever worry about how silly you might look or what people might think of you while doing your exercise. It's what you look like when you're dressed up and going out that counts, and you're going to look so fantastic after all this exercise that you'll forget all about appearing silly.

Your beauty routine tonight
Eyebrows and other facial hair
Don't ever be embarrassed about having facial hair. Women tend to treat the subject as something vaguely shameful, which is ridiculous. We all have facial hair, only it's more obvious on darker people. Dealing with it is simply another job to do like brushing your teeth or washing your neck.

If you have a bad problem with hair on your upper lip, electrolysis is the obvious answer. However, it is costly, you can only have a little done at a time and there might not be a salon near you. The inexpensive and effective alternative is either waxing, or depilation with a proprietary cream product.

Don't shave your upper lip. It doesn't do any harm, but the regrowth tends to be bristly.

If you've never plucked or shaped your eyebrows before and you have an unsteady hand, do take professional advice about getting it right. It could be a disaster if you plucked out all the wrong hairs, then tried to even yourself up and ended up with two different-shaped eyebrows! And if you choose the wrong shape you can give yourself a strange expression.

If you have never plucked before, and take the view that your eyebrows have always looked fine *au naturel*, take another look. One of the problems of getting older is the crêpiness of the skin on our upper eyelids, and if you also have a mass of stray hairs the combined effect could be dreadful. You'll look as if you have twice the number of lines on your eyelids when in fact it's all hair. An added problem is the addition of eyeshadow to the loose skin and hairs, and you soon end up with a smudgy, dirty-looking mess above your eyes, which is at odds with the endless trouble you have taken to look your best.

By employing a little judicious hair removal you can avoid all that. And it's so easy.

You will need
- hair band or grips
- cleansing lotion
- face flannel
- depilatory cream
- cotton-wool pads
- toning lotion
- tweezers

1. Start by tying your hair well back from your face and securing with a band or grips, or put on a bath cap.
2. Cleanse your face of all make-up. Wash and pat dry.

3. Fill your bathroom basin with water, which should be as hot as you can stand. Soak your flannel for a few seconds, then wring out.

4. Place the flannel over your face and press down. It should feel almost too hot to bear. Hold for twenty seconds or so, steep in the hot water again and repeat the process. This opens your pores beautifully and leaves the skin primed for hair or blackhead removal.

DEPILATION

Apply a thin strip of depilatory cream to your upper lip. Follow the instructions on the tube for the length of time it should be left.

EYEBROW PLUCKING

1. Plucking commences between the brows. Use a magnifying mirror on a stand, to leave both hands free.

2. Soak a cotton-wool pad in toning lotion. This is used to wipe over the area after a few hairs have been plucked out.

3. With your tweezers in one hand, use the thumb and fingers of the other hand to stretch the skin gently around the area you are plucking.

4. Proceed as quickly as possible, wiping with cooling lotion as you go.

5. Remove all stray hairs and space the inner corners evenly.

6. The shape of the eyebrow is formed by removing hairs *below* the brow, plucking in the direction of the growth, and supporting and stretching the skin with the other hand.

7. Stray hairs above the brow and at the temple may be removed as long as they do not form part of the main eyebrow growth.

8. If your eyebrows are extremely heavy, I suggest you follow this procedure over two or three sessions, as a totally new look will take some getting used to. Remember, you can always do a little more. If you take out too many hairs, they can't be put back! Over-plucked eyebrows should be allowed to grow and be kept tidy until sufficient hair has grown to form a new line.

When you have finished, wipe the plucked area over once again with toner, then rinse off the depilatory cream on your upper lip.

Although only a minor beauty treatment, eyebrow shap-

• • • • • • • • • • • • • •

ing can be an extremely important part of your overall grooming routine, as neglected eyebrows indicate a lack of care and attention to detail which could reflect poorly on you. I have also seen plenty of girls who have been transformed by taking charge of their eyebrows, and in particular it can add sophistication to what was once a 'little-girl' appearance.

Feeling hair-free is wonderful. If my eyebrows need plucking I feel that the whole world is gazing at the space above my eyes in horror, so take five minutes to get to grips with this essential part of your Fabulous in a Fortnight routine.

> **TIP:** *If the eyebrow-shaping procedure takes longer than you anticipated, wash off your depilatory cream. You don't want to forget it and have a rash!*

Checklist

1. Have you checked your shoes for scuff marks or worn heels? Even if they've been put away in boxes they are probably dusty, so don't leave it until the last minute to give them another polish.

   If your shoes are new, check that price tags have been removed!

2. If you've bought a new belt to go with a skirt or trousers, check that it'll fit the loops provided.

3. How's the length of that hem? You might have felt fine in it last year but you may have changed your ideas since then. If it's too short you'll feel like mutton dressed as lamb, too long and you'll feel matronly. Most of us have done running repairs and alterations at the last minute – I've even tried to let down a hem and press it while my husband was sitting outside in the car with the engine running!

I once had a favourite dress, a candy-striped affair with a sailor's collar. It gave me faithful service year after year and people always complimented me on how I looked in it. Then one day I went to a tennis party in it and caught sight of myself when I wasn't expecting to. I was shocked. I was the same weight and figure size I'd always been but in a split second I realized my face had got too old for the dress. Don't let yourself become a laughing-stock!

Be honest with yourself. It can work both ways. Are those trousers ageing? Is it the fabric, or the cut? Maybe you've just moved on a bit since those businesslike jackets, and yearn for a more fun look. When we spend half our lives wishing we looked older and were taken more seriously, and the other half striving to look younger and be thought of as 'with it', there's got to be a halfway mark when one becomes the other. There can be many changeover periods, and you might be the sort of person who swings from one mood or type of company to another.

Think about whether the clothes you loved last year give out the right message this year. Remember, you've moved on!

Maybe you only need to do some alterations? Cutting off the sleeves, replacing the buttons and removing lapels are just three of the inexpensive alterations I've had done recently, which have given two dresses and a jacket a further year or two of wear when I was going to throw them out. Try it.

This is the end of your fourth day and I hope you're keeping up with the diet and exercises. Please don't give up. Don't cheat, either. If you go out and see some wonderfully slender girl lapping up an iced doughnut with her coffee and wish you could be as lucky as she is, you will be! She's not lucky, nobody is. If she ate too much, she'd be fat like anyone else, so think ahead to the time when you'll have reached your goal weight, then it'll be just a matter of maintenance and you'll be able to eat doughnuts too. *You will*!

Your Meals for Day Four

BREAKFAST
1 scrambled egg
1 slice wholemeal toast *or*

25 g/1 oz Special K cereal
150 ml/5 fl oz skimmed milk

100 ml/3½ fl oz fresh orange juice

MID-MORNING
1 digestive biscuit
tea or decaffeinated coffee

MAIN MEAL
Salmon with Mashed Potatoes and Green Vegetables (page 180)
or
Pasta Primavera (page 184)

fromage frais with stewed fruit

LIGHT MEAL
Waldorf Salad (page 211) *or*
Smoked Chicken and Pesto Pasta Salad (page 203) *or*
1 round egg mayonnaise wholemeal sandwich

orange and grapefruit segments (tinned will do)
plain yogurt (optional)

SUPPER
25 g/1 oz porridge

Day Five

You are nearly at the end of the first week of your 'Fabulous in a Fortnight' plan, and I hope you're getting on well.

You should have lost a few pounds by now, but the main difference you should feel is *inches* slimmer. Many overweight people say that diets don't work. This is completely wrong. Diets *do* work. What they mean is that either the type of diet they've been following doesn't work, or they couldn't stick with a diet. I'm not criticizing anyone who loves food and finds it hard to control their eating, but dieting doesn't mean cutting your food intake right down and missing meals. Your diet is simply what you choose to eat and your pattern of eating. People who are overweight have usually got something wrong in the equation, and ideally, diets should be individually designed for the person concerned so that everything can be taken into account.

People who genuinely love their food never eat a lot. Plenty of food-lovers form clubs and societies and regularly meet at different restaurants to savour new tastes in food. True wine-lovers don't drink to staggering drunkenness. They take pleasure in savouring the wine, they love food and drink and don't have a problem with it.

The problem begins when food becomes an obsession, and it becomes an obsession out of a kind of hatred. Obsessive eaters rarely notice what they're eating. They'll eat very little in public, saving their binges for quiet times alone. They say diets don't work because food isn't being eaten for its own sake. It's filling a gap. Rather like smokers who wonder what to do with that yawning gap after a meal, dieters don't know how to fill the time if they're not eating. 'I can't have a cup of coffee without a biscuit,' said one of my clients. 'I can't sit watching people eat a pudding and not have one myself,' said another. Why not? It's not the biscuit or pudding they're missing. Eating can become a habit, and we programme ourselves so that coffee means biscuit, television means chocolate and a drink, shopping at the supermarket means squash and a cake for the kids.

I'm not totally against this. When I was little, my swimming lesson on a Saturday meant a stop at a café afterwards for a meringue. We all love our little rituals and they make life more interesting. They only stop being enjoyable when they're a habit. If part of being overweight is that routine of coffee and cake or telly and chocolate, *BREAK THE CYCLE!!*

Think yourself into a new person

Thinking yourself into a whole new persona is one step, and getting your diet right is another. You can't change yourself overnight but you can start by cutting three biscuits down to one, or making one helping of pudding last out so you don't need a second go.

My diet plans are always based on the understanding that slimmers aren't second-class citizens, and if everyone else is eating a biscuit or pudding, they can too. 'Have some fruit instead' is the usual advice for dieters at dinner parties, or 'Ignore the peanuts and choose the carrot and celery sticks instead.' Well, it doesn't sound much of a life to me. Vegetables and mineral water can be dressed up to sound thrilling, but we all know they're boring. When you see people in party frocks pulling into the twenty-four-hour service stations, it's not to buy petrol, it's to stoke up on the vast quantities of chocolate, crisps and nuts they've spent the last five hours trying to avoid, and in the process had a thoroughly rotten time.

• • • • • • • • • • • • •

I only ever recommend banning something on the grounds of spoiling your looks, as in the case of fried foods and chocolate, or for health reasons. Coffee, alcohol, fried foods and sweets are fine in small quantities, but we rarely stick with small amounts. Coffee and alcohol are addictive drugs which cause free radical attack (see the nutrition section, page 43), sweets contain too much sugar and give you spots, and fried foods contain far too much fat and also damage your skin.

Apart from this small list, banning foods doesn't work. *Restricting* yourself to small portions does; rationing yourself to so much a week and no more also works. Treating yourself well and allowing yourself proper, decent food like everyone else also contributes to lasting success.

The reason I mention all this is because today's meal choices include a delicious lemon caper sauce and a watercress sauce, both of which are pretty rich. I pondered over whether to reduce the calories by removing the cream and halving the butter, then I thought – why? They'd become completely different sauces, and I don't want that. So instead of having the full quantity, and ladling on huge amounts of insipid, calorie-free, boring sauce, which does nothing for the main ingredient and indeed detracts from it, why not have a couple of tablespoonfuls of something delicious and rich and tasty? Your slimming recipes are exactly as they were intended, and the good news is that you'll still lose weight. I promise.

Today and every day you can eat what slim people eat – only not too much. *Please*!

Foot and leg exercises

Ankles and legs are not what they were. Women used to take pride in having slim ankles and well-shaped calves, shown to advantage in high-heeled shoes, but the modern trend for exercise has led to over-developed calves and thicker ankles. Feet are designed for a great deal of movement, yet we let them sit in shoes all day or evening,

• • • • • • • • • • • • • •

immobile for hours. Try to get into the habit of doing these exercises every single day, when you are watching TV, sitting at your office desk, or even waiting for a train!

Foot flexing
Sit barefoot on an upright chair and cross one leg over the other. Stretch the toes downwards as far as they will go, pointing towards the floor. Stretch the foot back towards you until you can feel the pull on the front of the leg. Do six times, then change legs and repeat.

Foot circling
Still sitting in the same position, point the toes of the uppermost foot and draw six wide circles in the air, slowly. Reverse the direction and do six more. Change legs and repeat.

Joint stretch
Stand upright and take your weight on to one foot. Raise your other heel and bend your toe joints at right ankles so you are right up on your joints. Hold this position for a count of five, return the foot to the flat position and repeat three more times. Change feet and repeat.

Shake out
Standing on one leg, raise the other leg and loosely and vigorously shake the foot for a few seconds. Change feet.

By giving yourself a weekly pedicure and doing your foot exercises, you will soon have feet you can be proud of. Never forget that you could be called upon any time to reveal all, and if you suddenly twisted your ankle it would be a shame if some Good Samaritan stripped off your shoes and stockings to reveal appalling feet! Nice feet are worth the trouble, and knowing they're nice will give you confidence.

• • • • • • • • • • • • • •

Your beauty routine for tonight
Your feet

Feet generally don't get the attention they deserve. Neglected in favour of hands, encased for much of the year in tights, stockings or socks, they can become tired, sore and a potential health problem.

If your feet are in serious need of attention, I do advise that you go and see a chiropodist to get them sorted out. Don't be afraid or ashamed of your feet. Whatever they look like, however ugly you think they are, you can be sure that he or she has seen far worse. Hard skin on your heels and toes is a particular problem which you must get seen to, bad toenails are another. If, however, your feet are simply suffering from general neglect, or if you usually go to a salon and have decided to save some time and money doing them yourself, here's your step-by-step guide.

The good thing about this is that you don't have to put on your shoes afterwards and tramp home in the cold and wet. As soon as you've completed your massage and polished your toenails, you can put up your feet and relax with a nice drink!

This treatment takes about twenty minutes.

You will need:

- small nail scissors
- emery board or nail file
- cuticle remover
- bowl of warm, soapy water
- towel
- cotton bud
- cuticle oil
- exfoliating grains or sisal mitt
- hard skin remover or pumice stone
- scented body or foot softening lotion
- talcum powder
- nail varnish

1. Clip your nails first, before soaking, or they will become too soft. Make sure you cut straight across the nail in a line, not into the corners.
2. File to smooth the nail edges.
3. Apply a little cuticle remover to each nail, and put your feet in the bowl of warm water to soak for about five minutes.
4. While you are doing this, try giving yourself a hand and nail massage.
5. Remove one foot from the water. Using a cotton bud, gently work round each cuticle to remove dead skin. Do not dig under the cuticle as this can cause damage and fungal infection. Rub on a little cuticle oil.
6. Repeat with the other foot.
7. Using your exfoliating grains or sisal mitt, massage each foot well for a minute, until both feet feel thoroughly clean and surface dead cells have been removed.
8. Now take your hard skin remover or pumice stone, and work thoroughly on the heels and other areas of the foot which might have hard skin build-up. Rinse thoroughly in clean water.
9. Using your softening body or foot lotion, massage the feet for about a minute each. Use firm movements.
10. Apply talcum powder between the toes to prevent infection.
11. If you are varnishing your toenails, wipe each nail carefully with cotton-wool pad soaked in water or toner, to remove cream or lotion which could prevent the nail varnish staying on.
12. Following the same instructions for varnishing your fingernails, start with a base coat, and allow to dry.
13. Apply two coats of your coloured varnish. Allow to dry.
14. Apply a top coat. You should not put on your shoes for about half an hour.

Checklist

1. Have you checked your menus for the weekend? You have Sunday off, but you might need something for tomorrow and Monday.
2. Do you need anything in the beauty line? Cotton wool? Tissues? Make a note now.

Your Meals for Day Five

BREAKFAST
25 g/1 oz porridge *or*
2 slices wholemeal toast
butter from allowance
1 teaspoon marmalade or jam

100 ml/3½ fl oz fresh orange juice
tea or decaffeinated coffee

MID-MORNING
150 ml/5 fl oz skimmed milk
1 digestive biscuit

MAIN MEAL
Cod in Lemon Caper Sauce with Lime Rice
(page 179) *or*
Linguini in Creamy Watercress Sauce (page 185) *or*
¼ vegetable quiche with French beans and potatoes

fromage frais with stewed fruit or compôte (bottled will do)

LIGHT MEAL
egg mayonnaise salad *or*
1 jacket potato with prawns *or*
1 round wholemeal egg sandwich with watercress

mixed fruit salad

SUPPER
plain yogurt with sultanas and 15g/½ oz mixed nuts or flaked
almonds

NOTE: *Your main meal today can be a shop-bought quiche.
Despite the calorie content of the pastry in quiches, you only need
a quarter of a normal family-sized pie to make a satisfying meal,
and the recommended vegetable quiche for today contains 239*

• • • • • • • • • • • • • •

calories per slice. Add 175 g/6 oz potatoes and either vegetables or salad, and you have a filling and satisfying meal containing about 420 calories.

If you prefer a fish or bacon quiche, the calorie counts aren't going to vary very much, as long as you stick with the quarter portion. If you are very hungry and would like one-third of the quiche, the calories for your meal are approximately 500.

Day Six

With any luck, if you don't work at the weekend, you'll have a little more time to devote to your exercise today. And can you manage without your make-up today, to give your skin a breather?

Your meal plan is lighter today, to take into account that you might want to eat more tomorrow, which is a day off the plan. If you are spending Sunday with family or friends, it's difficult to keep to your diet, and in any case, Sunday lunches and teas are most enjoyable and won't do you any harm as long as you don't go mad!

Try also to get some good sleep. Sleep is one of your best beauty aids, and it costs nothing.

Your exercises today

Go back to the exercise section (pages 50–68) and try to get a full session in this morning.

If you've been doing the exercises every day, you'll see and feel some improvement by now, especially if you haven't done this sort of thing before. Toning exercises are vital to your figure. Most women feel that aerobic exercise does them the most good because it's exhilarating, and you need that kind of heart-pumping exercise to keep you healthy. It won't, however, change your shape. The best way to exercise is to *combine* aerobic exercise, muscle-toning and stretching.

Muscles need to be lengthened and strengthened and stretched for a good result to be seen in your shape. However much you feel you lack motivation when exercising at home on your own, you must keep it up. Get a video so you don't feel alone, or get a friend in. Go to a class if you need people around you or an instructor offering encouragement. Organize sessions at your place of work, or the local school. Above all, never neglect your toning exercises, *twice a day in the future*. The Fabulous Woman always exercises, but never to obsession. The Fabulous Woman owns her body, and never lets it get out of control. Are you becoming a Fabulous Woman yet?

Your beauty routine tonight
Posture practice and trying on your clothes
If you are going out tonight, you won't have time for more than getting yourself all spruced up, but of course if you are bathing you'll have time for a nail soak and a good massage with scented body lotion.

Set aside five minutes and practise your posture (page 24). This is especially good if you are going out and want to look at how you sit and stand in your party clothes. If you have a full-length mirror, try it now.

1. How do you look when holding a glass, cup or plate? Check what you are doing against the picture on page 28.
2. Fetch a low chair, similar to the depth of a sofa, and sit down on it. Do you look ungainly? A familiar problem is where your skirt is so tight, and your chair so low, that you have to splay your legs like a giraffe to get up out of it. There's nothing worse than heaving and straining to stand up, and you feel such a fool. By practising now, you'll learn how to wiggle to the edge and get your balance before standing up. See page 27.
3. Try sitting on an upright chair. Now cross your legs at the knee. Does anything show? Does this make your thighs look fat? The trick is to cross your legs at the ankles and bend the legs to one side. This *always* looks elegant.
4. Are you sitting up straight? Your chest needs to be raised, then even if you are leaning backwards and resting against the chair, you won't look sloppy or slumped. See pages 26.

• • • • • • • • • • • • • •

5. Are your clothes 'wearable'? Do straps stay on your shoulders, do the sides of your bra show when you raise your arms?
6. Is your bra visible under your top? Do you want it to be?
7. Is your skin up to being shown? If your dress is sleeveless, are your arms OK? If it plunges, how's the skin on your chest? *BE HONEST!*

Checklist

1. If you're planning to wear nail polish which you've had for some time, check that you can still open the bottle, and it hasn't become too thick. Nail polish lasts for so long that it can be a surprise to realize just how long it's been sitting in the drawer.
2. Check the colour match.
3. Have you any pins holding things up which you might have forgotten about? Maybe you did a hasty repair last time? Double-check.

Your Meals for Day Six

BREAKFAST
½ grapefruit or 100 g/4 oz tinned segments
1 slice wholemeal toast
butter from allowance
1 teaspoon jam
tea or decaffeinated coffee

MID-MORNING
2 Rich Tea biscuits
tea or decaffeinated coffee
mineral water

MAIN MEAL
Seafood Pilaff (page 181) *or*
Vegetable Chilli with salad (page 188) *or*
Herb Omelette with mixed salad and boiled potatoes (page 187)

Rice Pudding (page 215)

• • • • • • • • • • • • •

LIGHT MEAL
Warm, Spicy Chicken Salad (page 199) *or*
baked beans on toast *or*
1 round light cream cheese and grape wholemeal sandwich

2 pieces of fruit *or*
mixed fruit salad

NOTE: *If you have your light meal in the evening and are not going out, have an extra snack about 9 p.m. of a bowl of Bran Flakes or 2 Ryvitas with Marmite. Don't forget your daily six glasses of water.*

Day Seven

After six days, you need a day off! Staying on diets for weeks on end means that boredom soon sets in, especially if you've been restricting food and drink which you normally take with abandon. Never be too hard on yourself, but learn your limitations. Life really is too short to spend it denying yourself a bit of pleasure, but on the other hand, it's also too short to spend hating the size of your thighs or the roll of flab round your middle.

Some people are better than others at certain things. If you grind your teeth at the fact that some women stay slim effortlessly, comfort yourself with the fact that someone probably envies you your thick hair or strong nails. It may be that you'll have to battle with your weight all your life, but so be it. Don't make yourself miserable about it, find a way of dealing with it.

I don't actually think that food is a treat if it makes you feel fat, but if you can handle them, 'treat days' are a good idea and keep you in control of your figure. For instance, I have a client who's a professional dancer working Monday to Thursday, so she eats a high-carbohydrate, high-protein diet on those days and goes easy on salads, sweets and fruit. Friday feels like a holiday, so she has a light fruit lunch and goes out for a curry or Chinese meal in the evening. Saturday is her sweets day, so it's either a bar of chocolate or a packet of toffees while watching television, with salads and fruit for the rest of the day. Sunday is normal roast lunch day, then it's back to her strict regime for the next four days. This way she never feels she's missing out, her diet is sensibly balanced and varied and she stays slim.

Why not try to devise a regime for yourself which designates a day to foods you can't live without, such as a slice of rich fruit cake or a plate of chips, and a day to slightly stricter living, when you know it'll be no effort? But remember the rules. Don't have days of fasting. Don't have 'liquid only' days. Always eat regularly and eat small portions.

Some women have weight problems all their lives. It's easy to say don't get fixated by your weight, but that's because a fixation becomes an obsession and then you can't see the wood for the trees. Most people who worry obsessively eat too little. I can promise you from long experience that the secret of being slim is to eat regularly and healthily, and not spend time worrying and weighing everything. Relax. You have another week to go in your 'Fabulous in a Fortnight' plan, and you're going to look wonderful.

Day Eight

As soon as you've done your wake-up stretches and exercises, it's time to weigh and measure yourself to see how well you've done in the past week.

1. Turn back to page xx, write in today's measurements and compare them.

2. Have you lost weight? Are your measurements smaller? If not, do you know why? Have you cheated on the diet, or not done enough exercise?

3. If you have lost a few pounds – and a few pounds is all we're looking at – you'll feel pleased and eager to continue. If you haven't, the answer is NOT to eat less, although you can reduce the size of your portions just a little. You should still eat at the same times. Never cut out meals. Never change your regular eating pattern. It confuses your body which then stores fat at a faster rate. This diet is already calorie-restricted, and you should never go below your basal metabolic rate of 1,450 calories a day. If you do, you'll find the weight piles back on when you start to reintroduce more food. This is never the right approach.

   The answer to speeding up your weight loss is to increase your output of energy by doing more exercise. Think about what you could do in the next six days to exercise more. Take a walk at lunchtime? Go to an extra keep-fit class?

   Don't be despondent. This diet will work, it just needs a bit of adjustment for your personal needs, that's all.

   If your weight isn't falling, kick-start it with more aerobic exercise.

4. YOUR BODY SHAPE

How are your measurements? What I'd expect to see by now is a noticeably flatter stomach and an inch loss over your hips and thighs. If you are generally happy with your weight but unhappy with your shape, increase your toning exercises. Don't do this by increasing the amount of time you spend at each toning session – do it by increasing the number of times you do each session in a day. So do three or four five-minute stomach exercise sessions instead of two.

5. YOUR SKIN

You should see an improvement in your skin. Don't forget, we're not trying to turn you into a raving beauty, though that would be nice. A good complexion is always commented on. A poor one is also noticed. A poor skin doesn't just show itself in spots – it can be seen to be dirty, grimy, unhealthy and 'thick'. What you should be starting to see by now is a more translucent, clean appearance to your skin, the result of exfoliating, deep-cleansing and plenty of fruit, vegetables and water in your diet.

6. YOUR NAILS

Unfortunately nails grow slowly, but by removing excess cuticle and trimming hangnails you can expose a lot of nail which was previously covered, making the nail as a whole appear longer. If short nails are your problem, they should look a lot better.

The effect of daily nail massage takes some months, but in a fortnight you'll have started a process which will be rewarding. A good manicure, to my mind, has the effect of making you use your hands in a more confident way, and if you usually spend a lot of time and nervous energy avoiding situations where your hands are on show, knowing that you don't have to worry about them any more is a blessed relief.

Your exercises today

Following the exercise plan might be getting repetitive and stale. Don't let this happen! I do the full set every day myself, and fifteen minutes isn't a lot of time to commit to your figure. Well done for keeping it up!

If you want to increase your exercise, *don't spend longer doing each set*. Instead, you should increase the number of times you do the set every day, perhaps from two to three or four.

The full set of floor exercises is contained in my video *Fabulous in a Fortnight*.

The biggest trouble with exercising at home is that you tend to stop when you feel like it. Motivation can be a real problem when you're on your own, so I suggest that if you can't see through the whole set of exercises, you set a timer for a period such as five, ten or fifteen minutes, and tell yourself that you can't stop until it rings. Or use a piece of music which you'll see through to the end.

Remember that exercising on a full stomach can make you feel sick, and doing stomach exercises either after a meal, or for too long a period, can actually damage your back. When you do a sit-up and you press downwards, the internal pressure of all your organs is potentially damaging to the discs in your spine, and if you also have a stomach full of food I don't need to describe the effect! This is why we turn over after a few minutes of stomach exercises and stretch our spines in the opposite direction to decompress the discs.

If any exercise hurts, stop at once. There's a difference between the normal effort of exercising and pain, which is your body's way of telling you that it's had enough. It isn't worth crippling yourself for a good figure, and it isn't very glamorous to appear at a party on crutches!

If you are very overweight and are finding the exercises difficult, please don't despair. A brisk walk or a swim will still have great benefits, and you'll be building up your strength and stamina gradually towards the day when you suddenly find the exercises not so hard after all. That means you're getting fitter. I can't tell you how many ladies I've come across over the years who came to my exercise classes overweight and unfit, and scared that they'd be laughed at. Often they just came to get out of the house. Then they found they'd lost a few pounds, their waistbands were a little looser and people were asking them if they'd lost weight. A few

• • • • • • • • • • • • • •

months later they'd be at the front of the class in a tight leotard, working up a good sweat and exercising fit to burst. It's so rewarding and such a pleasure when this happens.

I have often been challenged by cynics as to why I preach the message that women prefer being slim to fat. 'Surely people have the right to be the size they want to be?' I am asked, or 'How do you know it's better to be slim?'

I know because people tell me. I don't deny that people have the right to be the size they're happiest with, and I'm not interested in telling everyone they should be a size 10. I only become involved when someone asks for my help. There are thousands, possibly tens of thousands, of women who are extremely slim or underweight, but I don't know of any experts who make a living helping such people to gain weight. I am completely open to any suggestions when it comes to helping women feel better about themselves, and I have yet to find anyone slim who longed to be a size 16.

Don't ever give up. You can have the figure of your dreams and you *will* astound everyone. Just keep at it and give it time. I promise it'll happen for you, and you'll look simply fabulous.

Your beauty routine tonight

1. Tonight you have to go back to Day One and complete your full body scrub (page 84).
2. Before you start the procedure, apply a deep-conditioning treatment or hot-oil treatment to your hair, and leave it to become absorbed.
3. Remove any nail varnish.
4. Lie in a bath into which you have put some scented or emollient oil.
5. Run a razor over your legs and under your arms.
6. Shower off and wash your hair thoroughly.
7. Towel-dry and apply rich scented body lotion.
8. Check your eyebrows for stray hairs.
9. Style your hair.
10. If you have time to relax after this, warm up your pot of olive oil and soak each set of nails in it for five minutes.
11. Pat dry with tissues and massage each finger and nail bed.

Checklist

1. Are all your buttons sewn on? Do you have a spare in case one pops off during the day? And a small emergency sewing repair kit?
2. If you are taking a handbag which only comes out on special occasions, or an evening bag, check it now. You might have put it away correctly, but these things have a habit of getting squashed underneath something for months and coming out looking battered. Remember to put away handbags with newspaper stuffed inside them.
3. Is your handbag big enough for all your bits and pieces? A friend of mine spent half an hour putting things in and taking them out again in her efforts to close the clasp, but in vain. It was a tiny pink bag suitable for the minimum of kit, but she was trying to cram in her powder compact, spare tights, lipstick and eyeliner pencil, a bunch of keys, tissues and a mobile phone!

Your Meals for Day Eight

BREAKFAST
25 g/1 oz porridge *or*
2 slices wholemeal toast
butter from allowance
1 teaspoon jam

MID-MORNING
Banana Milkshake (see page 90, i.e. Meals for Day One)
tea or decaffeinated coffee

MAIN MEAL
Chicken Supreme with Basmati Rice (page 176)
mixed green salad *or*
Crunchy Seafood Gratin (page 182) *or*
grilled or roast chicken and vegetables *or*
Spiced Vegetable Triangles (page 193) with either green vegetables
and carrot batons or a watercress, rocket and lamb's lettuce salad

stewed blackberry and apple or fruit of your choice (tinned will do)
2 tablespoons custard or evaporated milk

• • • • • • • • • • • • • •

LIGHT MEAL
2 slices smoked salmon with 2 slices brown bread and salad n*or*
1 round of smoked salmon wholemeal sandwich *or*
1 round cheese and tomato wholemeal sandwich *or*
your choice from the salads section (pages 199–211)

fresh fruit

SUPPER (optional)
1 slice wholemeal toast
scraping of butter and Marmite
bedtime drink or tea or decaffeinated coffee

Day Nine

Thought for the day

A lovely smile is one of your best assets. However much time you spend on your looks, however many conditioning treatments you give your hair, however ravishing your skin, lips and figure, if you've got a hard face you might as well not have bothered. Some people actually cultivate an aloofness which masquerades as 'cool', but in the real world where we all need to make friends and influence people you need to be approachable. People find it hard to pluck up courage to speak to someone new unless they've been introduced, and paving the way by looking pleasant is helping you as much as it is helping them.

It works in all walks of life. Nobody wants to employ someone who looks as if they're going to go off the deep end at every small criticism. If you're new in a neighbourhood people will look at you first to gauge whether you're likely to welcome a knock on the door. Any man who's thinking of asking you out for a drink will consider first if it's going to be worth his while even trying, and however glamorous you look, a hard, unfriendly face isn't likely to encourage him. It's hard to put on a cheerful face if you've got all the troubles of the world on your shoulders, but looking pleasant is as easy as looking miserable, so practise your smile. You're building your assets up as you go along, and most of these come for free.

A smile costs nothing. Make the most of the assets which

are the most easily acquired. Practise your smile. It isn't silly to suggest that you have someone photograph you in different friendly poses if you're really unsure of your best look. After all, you try on combinations of clothes, fiddle with your hairstyle and experiment with new ways of using make-up, so why not have a go at practising your facial expressions?

Your beauty routine tonight

We've already dealt with the first step, which is to get your skin into prime condition, and now we deal with make-up

Make-up

Make-up takes practice. Even when you've got it right, you need to revise and update your look from time to time. Age, a different hair colour or cut, weight changes and hormonal fluctuations can all affect the appearance of your make-up, so don't get stuck in a time warp. Always be open to experimenting.

THE PURPOSE OF MAKE-UP

Make-up is an art form, which reflects your mood and personality. Once you have mastered the basic techniques of colour blending and application, you can use your skill to create the look of your choice.

Most of us have used make-up to hide flaws at some time in our lives. Puffy eyes, shadows, the unexpected spot or raging thread veins are all easily covered up with make-up, and for sheer peace of mind and a psychological boost, you can't beat a layer of foundation, a lick of blusher and a bright dash of lipstick. But papering over the cracks can't last. Make-up should enhance your features and work with them, to create the best possible effect. If people are aware of your make-up rather than your face, either your skin is poor or not well primed in the first place, or you have used the wrong type of product. Anyone, even with perfect skin, can end up with a bad result simply because she used the wrong type of base.

'BUT I NEVER WEAR MAKE-UP!'
Make-up is not intended to create a mask which hides your skin. If you are blessed with a good skin, you are young, and have looked after your face since your early teens, you will be able to go without foundation quite happily. However, you might like to buy a tinted moisturizer for days when you have a few little blemishes, something none of us can manage to avoid.

Make-up doesn't block your pores or damage your skin. In fact when it is applied correctly to thoroughly clean skin it acts as a barrier to outside pollutants, and as long as you adhere to the golden rules of not leaving it on your skin for more than twelve hours, and cleaning off every trace, make-up will only serve to protect and enhance your complexion. Use *mascara* and a little *tinted lip gloss* for evening wear. Rather than clogging your lashes and colouring your lips, these products simply define what you've already got, and maintain a dewy, glossy and healthy appearance.

KNOW YOUR SKIN TYPE
The first step in good make-up technique is to know your skin type.

Skin type	Choice of foundation
dry and mature	cream or moisturized emulsion
dry and sensitive	cream or oil-based
combination	liquid, semi-liquid, all-in-one
oily	non-oily, astringent or water-based cake or block type
blemished	medicated liquid or block
allergic/sensitive	hypo-allergenic (with all known irritants screened out)

• • • • • • • • • • • • • •

STEP-BY-STEP PROCEDURE

1. Always start with a full cleanse, tone and moisturize.
2. Tinted foundation should be chosen to match your skin colour. To test, apply a small amount on your jawline. It needs to blend in with the colour of your neck. NEVER choose foundation to add colour to your face. It is a base, of a neutral, matching colour, and colour will be added to it.
3. Cream products can be applied with the fingertips. Never drag across the face or rub in. Application starts at the throat and works upwards, swiftly.
4. Liquid foundations should be applied with a sponge. Block and cake products should also be applied with a damp sponge.
5. Never use too much powder as it sets in fine lines. The best type of powder to use is loose, translucent powder. Apply with a ball of cotton wool, pressing it into the areas likely to become shiny, such as the sides of the nose, chin and lip. Using a large soft brush, gently and swiftly flick away the excess.

EYE MAKE-UP

Lining the eyes is a fashion which swings in and out of favour. According to the fashion at this time and your personal preferences, use eye-liner with care. Use of liner can appear to open, lengthen or emphasize the eye, depending on the area of application and the colour you've chosen. Accentuating the eyes with a soft pencil has become more popular as it gives a softer effect. Whichever you choose, you need to practise.

If you are young and new to make-up, or you'd like to experiment, there is an excellent video available called *Make-Up in Vogue* by Karen May. It gives you an hour-long, step-by-step guide to choosing and applying make-up, and deals with the best way to create different effects. Here are some useful hints on playing with eye colour in order to make the most of the shape of your eyes, or the effect you want to create.

Do practise by shading each eye differently, then comparing the two. It can be very amusing and enlightening!

Small eyes

1. *Colour the entire lid with a bright but soft tone to make bigger.*
2. *Echo the brow line with a soft sweep of colour in a darker, harmonizing shade.*
3. *Accentuate the centre lid area with a more definite and slightly contrasting shade, blending in to give fullness to the lid.*

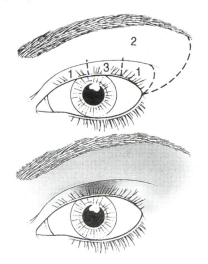

Overhanging lids

1. *Highlight the inner corner with a soft, light colour, and repeat under the lower lashes.*
2. *Shade the overhanging area very subtly to diminish its prominence. Use a matt eyeshadow, slightly deeper-toned.*
3. *Highlight the area under your brow, but do not use a frosted shadow. This deflects interest from the overhanging lid area.*
4. *Use a little eye liner if you wish, to emphasize the area closer to the lashes.*

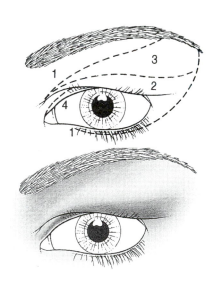

Prominent or heavy-lidded eyes

1. *Apply a dark shade of eyeshadow to the upper lid, close to the lashes.*
2. *Illuminate the brow-bone to take away interest from the prominent lids.*
3. *Mascara should be applied sparingly, just enough to define the lashes without drawing attention to the heavy lids.*

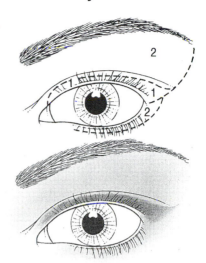

Close-set eyes

1. *The whole of the cavity of the eye should be brought forwards with a pale, soft eyeshadow, in a slightly oval shape.*
2. *A 'wing' of sweeping colour, slightly darker and brighter, can be taken from the centre of the eye, sweeping outwards.*
3. *An eye line in black or brown can be added or false eyelashes covering the outer third of the eye. The effect is to take interest to the outer corners of the eye.*

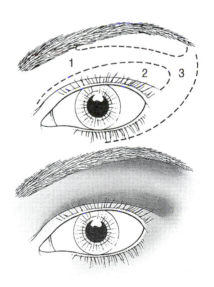

There are many other eye make-up techniques which can only be learned through trial and error, and I do suggest that you ask a friend for her honest opinion. I don't think we can be our own best judges. We see our own faces day after day and can't be objective. If you have nobody to ask, try different styles of make-up and you'll soon notice when people comment, although this can be quite depressing. Most of us have gone out at some time or another with a face we've spent ages on, only to be told we look tired and fed up, and the opposite is also true. Have you ever rushed out late after no more than a splash of cold water and a comb raked through your hair, only to be told you're looking well? It's just not fair, but then that's what being fabulous is all about!

Mascara

Who doesn't yearn for long, lustrous lashes? Trends in eyebrows may come and go, but when it comes to eyelashes the minimalist look will never be in fashion. Gorgeous lashes will always mean long and thick, and most women complain that theirs are too weedy.

Thirty years ago, the answer was to wear fake sable lashes – unbelievable though it might now seem – or at the very least fake natural hair lashes, and nobody worried that they were so obviously false. Nowadays the beauty houses prefer to market better mascaras which promise the earth, but can you do anything about your own lashes before you resort to artifice?

As with any hair, the condition of your lashes depends on good diet and the right choice of products you use on them. Time and care should be taken over the application of eye make-up, and especially over removing every trace at the end of the day. Each lash lives for about six months, but eyelashes break easily if not treated correctly. They need a break from make-up, and will become dry and drop out if they aren't cared for. After removing mascara, treat your lashes to a very light sweep of Vaseline every night, but avoid the eyelid or your eyes will be puffy in the morning.

1. Always make sure your mascara is fresh. After three months, throw old mascara away, especially if it has become lumpy and smells musty.

• • • • • • • • • • • • •

2. Curl your eyelashes with a professional curler before applying mascara. After curling, apply your first coat of mascara. To prevent smudges, do your lower lashes first.
3. Do the upper lashes, allow to dry, then apply a second coat.
4. Keep an old mascara wand handy which you have washed clean. Use this for a final separation of your lashes, and wipe clean again before you put it away.

LIPS

The intensity of your lip colour should be in balance and harmony with the rest of your face. Lip-liner and lipstick should never be obvious for their own sake. People should simply be aware that you have a nice mouth, and if your lips are the first thing people see when you come into a room, you've gone wrong. Why? Because if your whole look relies on one feature, you'll appear devastatingly different without it, and we all get caught out. The ideal to strive for is a look which is *enhanced* by such additions, but doesn't rely on them.

1. Always prime the lips first with a good moisturizer, and if possible, use a specialized lip-priming cream – Estee Lauder do a good one. This helps prevent lipstick 'bleeding' into fine lines.
2. Apply lip-liner, making sure you stay within the natural line of the lips. Going outside the line only works for photography and it can look ridiculous if it is obvious that you are trying to enlarge your lips. Remember, interest should always be taken upwards to your eyes, not down to your lips.
3. Apply lipstick with a brush, starting with the outline and then filling in the rest of your lips.
4. Blot with a tissue and apply a little more. The lipstick should always look as if it is part of your lips, not sitting on top of them.

BLUSHER

Blusher is another touchy area. Too much and you look like a clown, none at all and you'll look washed out. The wrong shade can suggest that you've either spent too long in the sun or just been caught raiding your son's money-box. Beautifully applied blusher, on the other hand, is a trick well worth acquiring as it can enhance and shape a face in a couple of short swirls.

Smile first before you apply blusher. Apply blusher to the 'apples' of your cheeks, and sweep gently up towards your hairline. Some people like to add a dash of blusher to their chin area, or forehead – again, this should be very subtle. Experiment with different shades of blusher by buying one of the products which offers several shades in one palette. This way you can choose from several alternatives, or mix them.

EYEBROWS

Finish your look with a little eyebrow colour which is softened with the side of a brush. At all costs, you must avoid a hard line. Choose a brush which has a comb on the other side, and make sure all your eyebrow hairs have been combed along their length.

Practice makes perfect. If you are getting ready for an occasion or party on Saturday (Day Thirteen), you aren't too late for a stunning new look, but you must spend time. Take into account the weather of the day and the light. If you are going to an evening event you can afford to be more generous and ambitious with colour; if you'll be out in the harsh daylight and likely to be screwing up your eyes against the sun, be very light with your foundation.

Above all, KEEP PRACTISING!

Checklist

1. Put on your outfit and check for underwear showing.
2. Check for visible panty lines.
3. Check for bra bulge.
4. If you are wearing stockings, double-check that you can sit down in your skirt and not have to keep tugging at your hem to hide the welts.
5. Don't rely on a jacket to hide a faulty dress or blouse underneath. The weather might change and be unexpectedly hot, or you might spill something and have to remove it. If all is not in order underneath you could be severely embarrassed.

Your Meals on Day Nine

BREAKFAST
25 g/1 oz unsweetened cereal (Rice Crispies, Special K, cornflakes)
150 ml/5 fl oz skimmed milk *or*
2 slices wholemeal toast
butter from allowance
1 teaspoon jam or marmalade

MID-MORNING
2 Ryvitas with cottage cheese or butter from allowance and Marmite

MAIN MEAL
Cauliflower Cheese and jacket potato (page 189) *or*
Chicken Biryani (page 176)

fromage frais with fruit compote (available in jars in good
supermarkets)

LIGHT MEAL
Salade Niçoise (page 201) *or*
1 round tuna wholemeal sandwich *or*
1 jacket potato
small tin baked beans
salad

small pot plain bio-yogurt with raisins and chopped walnuts

SUPPER
25 g/1 oz porridge
bedtime drink
mineral water

Day Ten

Why do we start every morning with a wake-up stretch by a window? Doesn't it seem a bit pointless?

Well, a wake-up stretch does exactly that – it wakes you up. When we're sleeping, our breathing is shallow, we're scrunched up into a ball more often than not, or we've been in one position for several hours. Stretching out feels good and the deep intake of oxygen into the bloodstream revives our sluggish system and makes us feel much fresher and wide awake, more quickly. So never ignore your wake-up stretch. Your muscles need it, and your circulation will also benefit.

How's the diet going for you? Have you found it hard or not so bad? The point is, can you keep it up for the future, and make daily exercise a part of your life too?

When you're young it's easy to think you've all the time in the world. A few months' lapse, gaining a few pounds, getting out of condition and a bit flabby . . . there's always the New Year, or next week. Well, it isn't like that. Ask any woman who's reached middle age and she'll tell you you're crazy to let your best years slip away like that. While you've got what it takes, take all you've got and make the most of it. I'm not saying it's too late in middle age, far from it. But youth is there to be enjoyed, and knowing that you look your best will not only help you get the best out of life but release a whole area of stress. So keep it up. You've only got four more days to go, and who knows what the new you will achieve? Go for it!!

Your teeth

While you're getting bathed and dressed this morning, spend a couple of extra minutes on your teeth. There's no time now for extensive cosmetic dentistry if your teeth don't look as you'd like them to, but a clean-up will work wonders. There's no excuse nowadays for teeth which aren't cared for, and a quick appointment with the hygienist might be a good idea if you haven't had a good clean for six months to a year. There's no shame in it. Regular brushing just can't shift everything, and if you're a tea or coffee drinker, or a smoker, brown stains tend to settle on the backs of your lower teeth, out of sight maybe, but not if you laugh uproariously at something!

Have regular check-ups too. You might not have problems, but old fillings can become leaky and this leads to food traps which can cause bad breath. And there's *nothing* a Fabulous Woman wants less than bad breath!

Other simple causes of bad breath are the following:

- going without breakfast
- stress and worry – they cause an acidic stomach
- strenuous exercise
- strict dieting
- eating garlic

The last cause is not thought by some to be a cause of bad breath, and it must be remembered that garlic is known to be good for the heart, but do take note that many people find the smell offensive, and you don't always know if foods contain garlic. Keep a general breath-freshening spray in your bag for emergencies, and check food-packaging labels for garlic content if an occasion is very important to you.

Strenuous exercise and missed meals lead to fat being burned, which while being exactly what you're hoping for, none the less lead to a by-product called ketones. Ketones are like exhaust in a car. The problem is that they also smell pretty foul, a smell we all recognize as similar to nail varnish.

This is another reason why my method of losing weight is based on eating regular small meals. You'll still metabolize fat cells, but not in an aggressive way, so you won't get bad breath.

Drinking plenty of plain mineral water also helps safeguard against bad breath; people who drink little usually have breath problems.

NOTE: *There are other causes of bad breath which are related to ill-health, so if you are worried, have a persistent problem and have eliminated the usual causes, see your doctor.*

Your beauty routine tonight
Hair

I don't know anyone who's happy with her hair. I know plenty of women who've settled for what they've got and given up worrying about it, but I don't know anyone who loves her hair. How about you?

If you have to get up early every morning to wash and style your hair, which won't go right until it's coated with anti-frizz mousse, styling gel and strengthening blow-dry spritzer, you're doing something wrong. If you then spend ten minutes with curling tongs, diffusers and velcro rollers, I'm surprised you've got time to go to work. And what if the wind blows?

You've got the wrong style. Maybe your cut is wrong, or your hairdresser hasn't advised you that your hair doesn't want to do what you want it to do, but you must get it changed. Life really is too short to spend half of it under the dryer, and though you might not believe it, there's another style somewhere that's right for you. Finding your best style requires professional help and experimentation.

Top hairdressers Toni and Guy give this advice:

1. Hair is under stress all the time from such environmental factors as:

- air pollution
- sun
- drying effect of wind
- air conditioning
- central heating or car heaters

Added stresses can be:

- too much washing and harsh shampoos
- colouring and perming
- build-up of hair products – sprays and gels, etc.
- hairdryers
- poor diet which doesn't promote healthy hair growth

The solution is to treat your hair well, and realize that it is a living structure which needs nourishing and looking after. Try these tips:

1. **Have your hair cut every six to eight weeks.**
   Even if going to a hairdresser's is an expense you find hard to manage, the best solution is a good cut. This way your hairstyle will last longer, and you won't need to make endless trips to sort out your style.
2. **Give yourself a conditioning treatment once a week.**
3. Help a style to last with a good setting mousse or styling spray.
   Apply styling agent at the roots of your hair. Allowing it to cover the hair shaft means that the weight of the product will drag your hair down and the style will be lost.
4. **Avoid '2 in 1' products of shampoo and conditioner combined.**
   They can cause a build-up on the hair, making it feel lank.
   Use a separate conditioner so you can decide where you want it to go – on the ends or on the roots.

Finally, don't be afraid to ask your hairdresser for a consultation. It is in their interest that you should be happy with the results, and time spent discussing your requirements is well spent for them as well as you. Having hair which looks after itself is a weight off your mind, so decide today to do something about it!

HOW DO YOU DEAL WITH FRIZZY HAIR?

Frizzy hair isn't helped by our damp climate. You need to coat the hair with a light serum to smooth out the cuticle. Frizzy hair tends to be rather dry, so a good moisturizing conditioner is important. After rinsing, rub a little extra conditioner over your hands, rub them together, then smooth over your hair – though don't do this on fine hair as it will make it lank.

Use a nozzle on your hairdryer and a medium heat. This way the air flow is concentrated where you need it, otherwise an open flow will make your hair fluffy. Follow the air flow down with your brush, which should be a wide, paddle-style brush.

WHAT CAN YOU DO ABOUT SPLIT ENDS?

You can't treat split ends, they have to be cut off. Prevention is the key, so don't use bristle brushes too often, don't brush too much, and avoid velcro rollers. Don't use too high a heat on your hairdryer, and comb wet hair starting at the tip and working an inch higher all the time to the root. Always use a good conditioner.

HOW CAN YOU GIVE LIMP HAIR A BIT MORE BODY?

You should use a specific volume-building shampoo, a separate conditioner and a mousse or spray gel. All products should be light in texture, as limpness is often caused by, or made worse by, the actual weight of the hair products themselves, which drag your hair down.

Use volumizing styling products on the roots, not the ends, and blow-dry from the roots out.

WHAT IF I GET A SUDDEN INVITATION, AND MY HAIR'S A MESS?

Always try to find time to wash it. Dry shampoos don't make you feel so fresh, and unless your hair is really long, you should be able to get a shampoo and blow-dry down to ten minutes at the most. If you haven't time, or you're at work, damp down your hair, use velcro rollers for a lift (you should keep some in your desk drawer), and finish with backcombing and sprays to hold style. It's a bit of a patch-up job, but it's better than doing nothing. Remember, if you're a true Fabulous Woman, your hair *always* looks nice and you're never caught out. Your hair should be freshly washed and styled every evening or morning so it always looks its best.

Checklist

Do think about your hair when it comes to going anywhere where it might be likely to be windy, wet or hot. If your hair is short, you won't have too much of a problem, but what if it's not?

You won't need me to remind you of some of the disasters which can strike your hairdo, or the effects of the wind, but here are a few reminders:

- A stiff breeze can whisk your hair across your face, catching on your lipstick. The result is long pink 'whiskers' across your cheeks!
- Your hair becomes matted and tangled.
- Your hair becomes greasy and lank over a period of hours when you are having to continually tug and smooth it back into place.
- It exposes parts of your face you'd rather remained hidden, such as your forehead or ears.

Your Meals for Day Ten

BREAKFAST
2 slices wholemeal toast
butter from allowance
1 teaspoon marmalade or jam *or*
25 g/1 oz cornflakes or Rice Crispies
150 ml/5 fl oz skimmed milk *or*
½ grapefruit

MID-MORNING
Strawberry Milkshake: blend 100 g/4 oz fresh strawberries or a
small tin of strawberries with 100 ml/3½ fl oz skimmed milk

MAIN MEAL
1 slice asparagus and salmon quiche or asparagus and cheese quiche
green vegetables
2 new potatoes *or*
Mexican Chilli Chicken (page 177)
colourful mixed salad

Poached Pears (page 214)

LIGHT MEAL
1 scrambled egg on 1 slice wholemeal toast *or*
1 jacket potato with egg mayonnaise
salad *or*
1 round egg mayonnaise wholemeal sandwich

fromage frais or natural bio-yogurt with 2 teaspoons fruit compote
mineral water

SUPPER
1 slice wholemeal toast
butter from allowance
Marmite or 1 teaspoon jam
bedtime drink

• • • • • • • • • • • • • •

Day Eleven

You're nearly at the end of your fortnight's plan, and I hope I have succeeded in showing you how significant an improvement you can achieve in such a short space of time.

At the end of the fourteen daily plans, I have included a selection of 'Famous Disasters'. Even if you aren't planning to go anywhere and are just using this book as a getting-to-grips-with-yourself improvement plan, the stories contained in this section are a cautionary reminder of what can go wrong, despite our best efforts. The women I talked to were all experienced social-eventers who still managed to make some wild errors of judgement and ghastly mistakes, so do read these amusing tales of woe.

Of course, it would be a shame if we went through life so terrified of putting a foot wrong, saying something out of place or wearing the wrong outfit that we either never went out of the house or remained steadfastly rigid and po-faced at social events. Part of life's natural dynamics are the learning processes we go through when we make a major gaffe, and people can love us because or in spite of them.

If you knew it all, you wouldn't be reading this book. Even people who think they know it all are just as likely to find themselves feeling like fish out of water, especially when faced with an occasion which is outside their normal circle or experience. Different levels of society have their own rules, an example being artistic gatherings as opposed to sporting get-togethers. Etiquette exists to ease us through these minefields, so that whatever the different conventions, a common thread of behaviour runs through them which enables the outsider to feel at ease. This is why certain rules exist. People may mock, but only by there being a common thread of manners and behaviour is it possible to slide effortlessly from one set to another without feeling embarrassed or out of place. The basis of good manners and etiquette is to make others feel at ease.

Don't ever get too hung up about an unfamiliar gathering. Someone is the host or in charge, and it is their responsibility to incorporate nervous guests and see to it that they are catered for. Just smile, which will encourage people to approach you, and look your best. *You can do no more.*

Your exercises

A quick recap on your exercises. It all depends on whether you're reading this book in the depths of winter or during the hopeful spring and summer months, when it's so much easier to get out and take more exercise. The wonderful thing about summer is that we get a 'second day'. You can work all day, come home and get changed, and set about several hours of a completely different activity outdoors. Gardening and walking are two activities which spring to mind, and not only do they improve your figure, they get you out of the kitchen and away from the delights of the biscuit tin.

Winter means sitting indoors – unless of course you're the type to go to the gym. It's hard to work up enthusiasm for fifty lengths of the pool when you know you're faced with a freezing walk back to the car park afterwards, but you can choose a different activity. Even staying at home can lend itself to exercising, and you won't be sorry. I've included the exercises in this book for just such a purpose, and they really work.

I appreciate that telling you to get out into the fresh air for a walk won't go down well with everyone. Some people simply hate being out of doors and the idea of tramping through fragrant woodlands fills them with dread. It's often the state it leaves their hair in, or the effect of the drying winds on their complexion, which I can understand. However, it's like taking your medicine, cleaning out your cupboards or finishing the ironing. The ends justify the means, and if you can spend your life having an enviable figure which everyone remarks on, your waistband feels lovely and loose and your thighs have daylight between them, a daily walk seems a small price to pay.

The same goes for your floor exercises. Yes, they can be boring. But what would you rather be, bored or fat?

Today, please try to go through the full set of exercises, which lasts for just fifteen minutes, twice or three times.

Your beauty routine tonight

Repeat the full manicure and pedicure treatments you did last week on Days Two and Five.

To save time, you will obviously be using the same set of tools for both hands and feet, and here is the best order to go about it:

1. Fill a bowl with warm soapy water. Clip toenails, apply cuticle remover and immerse both feet in the bowl. Leave to soak for five minutes.
2. File fingernails as before. Apply cuticle remover. Soak your left hand (if you are right-handed).
3. Remove one foot from the water and pat dry. With your free hand and using a pumice stone or rough-skin remover, remove all hard surplus skin from your foot. Repeat with the other foot.
4. With a cotton bud, remove excess cuticle from all your toenails.
5. Remove left hand from water and pat dry. With both hands, apply rich moisture lotion to your feet, massaging in thoroughly.
6. Raise your feet onto a stool or chair, to prevent the cream from staining or marking surfaces, and allowing it to be absorbed.
7. Working on the one hand, remove cuticles, clip hangnails and massage a small amount of cuticle oil or hand cream into the hand and nail bed. Soak the other hand.

• • • • • • • • • • • • •

8. After three minutes, repeat the full cuticle procedure on this hand. Massage in cuticle oil and hand cream, and massage both hands, paying particular attention to the base of your nails, for two minutes.
9. Do your foot and ankle exercises.

Your Meals for Day Eleven

BREAKFAST
2 slices wholemeal toast
butter from allowance
1 teaspoon marmalade or jam
tea or decaffeinated coffee
mineral water

MID-MORNING
1 banana

MAIN MEAL
Poached Cod or Salmon Parcel (page 180)
vegetables
2 mashed or boiled potatoes *or*
small vegetable pizza
colourful mixed salad

Baked Apple and Custard (page 213)

LIGHT MEAL
1 jacket potato with cream cheese and chives *or*
3 Ryvitas with cottage cheese and grapes *or*
2 pittas filled with mixed salad

pot of jelly

SUPPER
mixed fruit salad: 1 sliced banana, 1 apple, 1 pear, 10 grapes *or*
small tin fruit salad with 1 fresh sliced banana

• • • • • • • • • • • • • •

Day Twelve

Thought for the day: long- and short-term goals

I make no apologies for the fact that looking and feeling Fabulous in a Fortnight is a short-term goal. If I said Fabulous in Four Months most people would lose interest, and in any case, two weeks is not an unrealistic boast.

However, most people fail in their improvement programmes simply because all their aspirations for themselves are short-term. We want to fit into a wedding-dress, we want to look good for a party or a holiday. Then we slip back to our old ways. I've never been able to decide whether we're a nation of goal-driven people, unable to motivate ourselves beyond a concrete reason for looking good, or simply lack the discipline. One thing's for certain though: most people who lose weight successfully put it back on again, and people who are inclined to gain weight continue to do so.

Long-term goals tend to be more wishy-washy, hence the failure rate. Knowing you need to look good for a Millennium party is hardly going to get you dashing off to join the nearest gym or signing up for a series of massages and manicures at the local spa. There's always time, let's face it. Who needs three years to get ready?

I too have felt defeated, depressed and dreary about my looks and figure at some time or another. Having children and staying at home can mean no reason to look good, and I too know what it is to be severely discontented with your looks. Papering over the cracks became a part of my life, always carrying those extra pounds didn't matter because I'd discovered the art of dressing to hide them. My hair I gave up on and made a joke about. So what changed?

Funnily enough, it was talking to a relative who was forty years older than me. 'So how are you going to spend the next forty years?' she asked, and I felt myself go cold all over. 'Well, it's true that you might die next week,' she went on, 'but you could just as well live for forty or even fifty years more. How do you plan to fill the time?'

How indeed? How much longer was I going to put off my goals? Was I really going to spend half the time feeling dissatisfied with my hair and figure and the other half promising myself I'd do something at some indeterminate time? The children had grown, I'd got married again and settled. So what motivation was there left and, more importantly, with only one chance of a life, was this how I was going to spend it?

Life is not only too short, it is possibly too long also. Can you bear the thought of all this guilt over a piece of Christmas cake or hiding your stomach under a long jacket for another couple of decades? If a diet hasn't worked for you, find another one. Have you really worked hard for that flat stomach or smaller thighs? You know, for years I complained about my thin calves. 'No matter what I do,' I'd say, 'I can't get any shape into them.' Then I thought, 'But what do I do? I do exercises every day for a week, they hurt, so I don't do them again for three months. I haven't tried at all!' And I have clients like that. 'I've tried everything for a flat stomach,' said one recently, 'and nothing works.' But, you see, she hadn't tried everything, or at least she'd tried everything for a fortnight and then given up.

I can promise you that if you make something your long-term goal, set reasonable targets and stick with a plan you can fit into your life, you'll succeed. Long-term goals matter because if you have to walk this earth for three, four or five more decades, you might as well enjoy yourself. Typical changes you can make are:

• • • • • • • • • • • • • •

1. Stop smoking.
2. Only drink alcohol on a Saturday.
3. Say 'I don't drink' – you'll start to believe it.
4. Stop eating one type of food – such as biscuits – and never have them again.
5. Say 'On Monday and Thursday morning I have my walk' and make it compulsory. Of course you can do it – you go to work, don't you?
6. Do ten minutes of stomach exercises every day whether you want to or not.
7. Soak your nails in olive oil on Sundays and Wednesdays whether you want to or not.

You can make your own list, but the key is not to fit things in. You don't 'fit in' taking your children to school or going to work. Another fun way of doing it is to choose a date on your calendar – any day up to a year ahead – and simply writing in it 'Go for a five-mile walk' or 'Go to the pool for 100 lengths'. Then it's an appointment you have to keep!

Your beauty routine tonight

Fake tan

Have you ever used fake tan before? Why not have a try?

I remember self-tanning products coming out in the 1960s, and they were a revolution for the girls in my school who hadn't had a ritzy summer holiday abroad. Returning from a wet week in a windswept Welsh cottage, I recall panicking at the idea of going back to school and meeting my chums who'd spent a fortnight being tossed by the waves of the French Riviera, so it was with some desperation that I turned to Outdoor Girl's wonderful new product, Tanfastic.

For some reason I brazened it out when confronting my gaping classmates. I shall never forget the silent stares as twenty-five pairs of eyes ran slowly down my body, stopping to wonder at my orange-stained palms, and back up again to my face which looked like a burns victim. 'It was ever so hot in my back garden,' I stammered, and sank gratefully behind my desk-top. Self-tanning preparations were in their infancy, and so was I.

Suffice it to say that in the ensuing thirty years I've got to grips with the procedure and now consider myself a complete expert. And how the products have improved! No longer must your bedroom windows be left open all night to fumigate the place, and the colours are so good it's a waste of time even contemplating sunbathing. With all the furore over the dangers of ultra-violet light, not to mention the tangible ageing effects, I've been steadfastly pouring the stuff over myself twice a week for longer than I care to admit to, but remember that too deep a tan can also be unfashionable these days. For the busy girl who cares about looking old before her time, faking it is the only solution.

Follow these step-by-step instructions for a natural-looking gentle glow over your whole body:

1. Shower or bath and *thoroughly* exfoliate your body.
2. Make sure your legs are hair-free.
3. Pat yourself dry, and apply a *thin* layer of light body lotion, paying special attention to your knees, heels, tops of feet (in the bend of your foot), elbows, and any dry skin at the back of your shoulders. This layer of lotion must be very light. Rub in well and wait five minutes.

START WITH YOUR FEET AND LEGS

1. Take some self-tanning lotion (about the size of a 2p piece) into one palm.
2. Distribute evenly between both hands.
3. Put your left leg up on to a chair and start at your foot. Using 'mirror' actions, do wide circular movements with both hands, working both hands down your leg at the front and up at the back. Do not work lotion into your heels, under your feet or on to your toes. Rub in at this point to 'blur' the edges.
4. Run a finger quickly between each toe.
5. Take a similar-sized amount of lotion and continue upwards. Use wide, circling and sweeping movements, both hands in harmony with each other. Pause at your knee. With a dry tissue, rub over your knee, then sweep a hand over the area again.

• • • • • • • • • • • • • •

6. Continue upwards over the thigh. You need to be sure to get the lower part of your leg right first, as you don't want to get tanning lotion on your chest by leaning forwards on a thigh which has been 'done'.

Repeat on your right leg.

TRUNK AND ARMS

1. The same action should be used for both arms and your trunk, except that you can only use one hand to apply lotion to each arm.
2. Don't forget to rub the lotion into your elbows, rub roughly with a dry tissue and sweep your hand over the elbow again, lightly.
3. Remember the backs of your upper arms and under your chin, up to your jawline.
4. Use similar sweeping movements over your chest, covering as much of your breast area and abdomen as you choose.

FACE

You should use a special facial tanning cream, gel or lotion.

HANDS

Hands can be tricky, but after years of experimenting, I have found the perfect method of ensuring two evenly tanned hands with no stained nails!

1. Remove rings. Run a couple of inches of soapy water into your bathroom basin.
2. Using *your left hand only*, squeeze out a 1p-piece size of lotion on to your fingertips. Massage into the back of your right hand, making sure you blend in with the wrist and forearm.
3. Blend round the sides of your hand and down the fingers, stopping short of the nails.
4. Bend your fingers and rub the knuckles briefly on a towel to prevent the tanning lotion from settling in the creases.
5. Run a finger between each finger to remove any stray cream.

To remove lotion from your left hand, place your hand in the basin of water, swish around thoroughly and wipe dry.

Allow about ten minutes before you repeat the procedure on the other hand.

• • • • • • • • • • • • •

This all sounds complicated and time-consuming, but it isn't. Once you are practised it takes about five to ten minutes. Leave your clothes off for about twenty minutes if possible, to allow the lotion or cream to be thoroughly absorbed and prevent streaking, but thereafter the full colour should develop in about four hours.

Is it more trouble than it's worth? Not for me, it isn't. Compare this method of tanning with sunbathing or a sunbed session. It costs pennies per time. You need do the whole performance no more than twice a week, and at about ten minutes a time I think it's time well spent and saved. The finishing touch is that it protects your skin from damage, it avoids that dreadful leathery look which is inevitable for sunbathers when they get older, and it saves your life.

If you are not experimenting with fake tan tonight, do your body exfoliation or have a good invigorating scrub, as you don't want to be red and raw too near your important event. It's also a good idea to apply a facial mask again, and check on facial hair.

Your Meals for Day Twelve

BREAKFAST
25 g/1 oz Special K or two Weetabix
150 ml/5 fl oz skimmed milk
1 teaspoon sugar

MID-MORNING
1 pot bio-yogurt or fromage frais with sliced apple

MAIN MEAL
Salmon and Pasta Salad (page 202) *or*
Courgette and Tomato Gratin (page 190) *or*
Country Chicken Casserole (page 173)
dry-roast potatoes
carrots and French beans

Winter Fruit Salad (page 215) with fromage frais

• • • • • • • • • • • • •

LIGHT MEAL
Jacket Potato with Coronation Chicken (page 196) *or*
lentil soup and 1 crusty bread roll *or*
1 round salad wholemeal sandwich

2–3 pieces fresh fruit or mixed fruit salad

SUPPER
1 slice wholemeal toast
Marmite or 1 teaspoon jam
grapefruit segments
bedtime drink

Day Thirteen

You are nearly at the end of your 'Fabulous in a Fortnight' plan, and I do hope that you've enjoyed it.

At the beginning of this book I said that similar treatments at a health farm would cost you thousands of pounds. A top-to-toe day at a London salon costs about £250. So has it been worth doing all this for yourself?

Given the straight choice, with no expense spared and no arrangements to make, I daresay we'd all go for the health farm. The day at a salon is pretty acceptable too, so why not leave everything until the last minute and book yourself a day to do the whole lot in one fell swoop?

For a start, you can't speed up the process of losing weight. Second, while you can certainly feel fantastic after a day of plucking and tweezing, massaging and conditioning, you can't improve seriously neglected skin, nails and hair in one day. You'd just be papering over the cracks. If you looked so wonderful you wouldn't have bought this book, so presumably you're suffering from a little gentle neglect?

If you've been eating the wrong things it'll show in your skin. If you're tired it'll also show in your eyes and skin condition. You can't put that right in one day at a salon. There are no short cuts to beauty and a slim figure, but neither does it take for ever to make a significant difference.

This fortnight has been all about taking yourself in hand, and I hope you've also disciplined yourself to get plenty of sleep, stay off the alcohol and drink plenty of water. Yes, I think it's a bore not to drink. Yes, I think it's a bore to go to bed early with half a pound of cream on your shoulders and neck. But it's not permanent. This has been a rest cure, and you've taken yourself in hand. Please feel that this programme is here for you to take up any time you need it. It's not meant to be a permanent way of living because that wouldn't be realistic. It is important, though, to adopt a proper pattern of grooming which fits into your daily schedule, because being on top of little beauty chores means you'll never get caught out.

Your beauty routine will open doors for you, because by feeling beautiful, you'll radiate confidence.

Your beauty routine tonight

Tonight is a full recap. You will have got to grips with every bit of your body by now, so all you need to do is repeat everything.

1. Run a deep, scented bath.
2. Follow the full body and facial exfoliating procedure.
3. Shower off the soap or exfoliating cream. Shave underarms and legs.
4. Apply a facial mask. Lie in the bath for ten minutes.
5. Remove the mask, rinse thoroughly and dry off.
6. Apply your usual night moisturizer (or daytime moisturizer if you are doing this in the morning).
7. Apply body lotion and massage well.
8. Pluck eyebrows while your pores are still open.
9. Style your hair if you have washed it.

Checklist

1. Do you have tissues, cotton wool, etc., for emergencies?
2. Is your handbag big enough?
3. If it is going to be hot, your feet might swell. Do you need a refreshing foot spray if you have to stand for a long time?
4. Do you have some handbag-size handcream?
5. Do you need spare tights or stockings?

• • • • • • • • • • • • • •

6. Should you carry a spare set of make-up if the day will be a long one?
7. IS YOUR HANDBAG BIG ENOUGH NOW?!

Your Meals for Day Thirteen

BREAKFAST
25 g/1 oz porridge *or*
2 slices wholemeal toast
butter from allowance
1 teaspoon marmalade or jam *or*
1 boiled egg
1 slice wholemeal toast

tea or decaffeinated coffee

MID-MORNING
1 apple
1 pear
100 ml/3 ½ fl oz skimmed milk *or*
Banana milkshake (page 90)

MAIN MEAL
¼ bought chicken pie or whole individual chicken pie (see note)
2 tablespoons French or runner beans
carrots *or*
Spicy Chicken with Chilli-fried Red Rice (page 178)
vegetables or salad *or*
Spaghetti with Smoked Salmon, Dill and Watercress (page 184) *or*
Money Bags (page 186)
crisp mixed salad

Baked Banana Suzette (page 213)

LIGHT MEAL
2 scrambled or poached eggs
1 slice wholemeal toast *or*
Salmon and Corn Chowder with crusty bread (page 196) *or*
salad of your choice from salads section (pages 199–211)

mixed fruit salad

• • • • • • • • • • • • • •

SUPPER
2 slices wholemeal toast
butter from allowance
Marmite or 1 teaspoon jam
100 ml/3½ fl oz skimmed milk

NOTE: *Don't be put off by the fact that you are having pastry for this meal. I suggest you eat a small amount of the pastry and leave the bottom layer. Unless you are cooking for a family and it will therefore be worth making your own pie, it is a fiddly job which takes longer than the final enjoyment of the meal warrants!*

As with all meals on this diet, portion control is the key. If you keep to a small portion and supplement it with vegetables, you will have a nourishing, satisfying and speedy meal of around 375 calories, excluding vegetables.

By adding 100–175 g/4–6 oz boiled potatoes and a serving of greens your total calorie intake will be just 555 calories, perfectly acceptable for the main meal of the day.

Day Fourteen

You've reached the last day, so it's time to weigh and measure yourself again.

Check your findings against your chart (page 71). How do you measure up?

With any luck you've lost up to half a stone and several inches. Has it been easier than you thought? Didn't you think you had to eat a lot less in order to lose weight?

Your exercises

Do your exercises today as usual. Try to do an extra brisk warm-up session, to give you a healthy glow.

Your beauty routine

If this is a special day for you, you won't have left anything to chance or the last minute, and all you need to do is have a lovely scented bath, style your hair and either tidy up your nails or apply polish.

Remember to allow at least half an hour for your toenail polish to dry completely, or you could find that not only has it smudged, but your tights have stuck to it, and you'll end up tearing the fabric to remove them!

Your Meals for Day Fourteen

BREAKFAST
2 slices wholemeal toast
butter from allowance
1 teaspoon marmalade or jam *or*
25 g/1 oz cereal with 150 ml/5 fl oz skimmed milk

100 ml/3½ fl oz fresh orange juice
tea or decaffeinated coffee

MID-MORNING
Banana or Strawberry Milkshake (pages 90 or 147)

MAIN MEAL
Cashew Nut Korma (page 191) *or*
poached halibut or cod
plain steamed vegetables
2 mashed potatoes *or*
Kedgeree (page 183)

150 ml/5 fl oz Rice Pudding (page 215)

LIGHT MEAL
1 jacket potato
winter salad *or*
small tin spaghetti in tomato sauce
1 slice wholemeal toast
salad *or*
2 pittas filled with salad

SUPPER
1 Weetabix or Shredded Wheat
100 ml/3½ fl oz skimmed milk
low-calorie chocolate bedtime drink

Famous Disasters

Sometimes, despite our best efforts, a real disaster strikes. It might not seem so bad to others, but when you've spent time planning and preparing your appearance for a special event and it all goes wrong, the day can be ruined. I scoured the memories of some of my acquaintances and came up with some real cringers.

ANGELA, 46, is a sales negotiator
'I was out on a first date and was desperate to hook this man! We had soup for starters and I had a poppy-seed roll. After the dessert I went to the ladies and to my horror I saw that my teeth were full of little black poppy seeds, which looked absolutely dreadful. Obviously he knew what they were and wouldn't have thought it was my teeth which were bad, but the embarrassment came from knowing that he'd been looking at me laughing for a couple of hours, and these black teeth. It was even worse, going back to the table with him knowing that I'd cleaned my teeth. It didn't work out.'

VICKY, 22, is a hairdresser
'I was a bridesmaid, and I had this elaborate hairdo which was all piled up on top with a twirly bit. Although we practised doing the style beforehand, we didn't know what it'd be like on the day and it was a disaster. The top bit kept falling down round my face, and I kept pushing it back up. By the end of the day – and it was twelve hours – my hair

was in such a state from constantly pushing the top bit back up and trying to pin it, I looked a right mess. I wish we'd chosen something simpler!'

SYLVIA, 38, is a GP

'Shoes! I always wear them in, but on one occasion I didn't and my feet were on fire by the end of a couple of hours. I was hobbling, my heels were bleeding and my tights sticking to the blood! I feel pain just talking about it.'

JACKY, 31, works in a wine bar

'I was at a work party, wearing a low-cut dress. I was happy and sparkling and generally enjoying myself, then I felt something scratching my chest. I put a hand up and found the wire from under my bra was curling up, and when I caught sight of myself in the mirror it just looked like a huge insect had settled there. The problem was not knowing how to deal with it, so I just held my wine glass in front of it and rushed to the loo. My biggest embarrassment was wondering how long it had been like that!'

SALLY, 22, is a hairdresser

'I used to wear acrylic nails. Last Christmas my husband and I threw a big party, and at one stage I had to go and fetch another case of wine. I was opening it in the middle of all these guests, and had put my fingers under the cardboard flap to lever it up. My fingers slipped, my hand flew out and two of my nails took off across the room. At first everyone laughed, then there was silence, and those who hadn't seen it were saying, "What's happened?" and others were saying, "Oh, it's OK. Sally's nails have just come off!"

'I still feel I can't look people in the eyes. I've given up those nails and decided to do something about my own.'

MARION, 52, is a senior design engineer

'It was about ten years ago. There was an important meeting at work, a lunchtime reception to introduce senior staff to the parent company executives. It was a boiling hot day and I'd already become overheated travelling in my car, which had been parked for several hours in the full sun. To make matters worse, the room we were in was all glass, and simply boiling hot. I was holding a glass in one hand and a plate of food in the other, conscious that the perspiration was running down my back, and it was starting to break out on my face, too. Mind you, everyone was hot, but I always perspire heavily on my face.

'I grabbed a paper napkin, which was turquoise in colour, and every now and again I'd take a little dab at my cheeks and top lip. I chatted for an hour, feeling ghastly, then I went to the ladies room and to my horror I saw that my entire face was covered in tiny turquoise dots of paper! Why a kindly woman hadn't told me, I'll never know. The other problem was that I had to wash down my face, and I hadn't brought a scrap of make-up with me, except a lipstick, so I had to finish the entire meeting with a shiny face. I now carry a little bag of everything, just in case!'

SANDRA, 47, is a shop assistant

'My embarrassing moment was going to a Christmas drinks party with my sweater inside out. I'd bought it in a sale, and it was actually one of those "blue cross" items, you know, when they further reduce everything for a couple of hours to practically nothing. My label had three price reductions crossed out, and alongside the blue cross it said "to clear". I walked around with this showing for over an hour.'

PAULINE, 26, is a leisure centre instructor

'I went out with a roller in the top of my hair. Simple as that. I was meeting friends in the bar of this club, and it felt worse because I waltzed in a bit, sort of going "Dah-dah! Here I am!" Then a girl said, "Did you know you have a roller in your hair?" and I pretended it was done for effect, but everyone knew.'

• • • • • • • • • • • • • •

JANE, 21, has just been awarded her degree in fine arts
'I know this doesn't sound very embarrassing, but it was to me. You try and think of everything, but the day of my degree ceremony was terribly windy, a real gale-force. We were ages having the pictures taken, and my hair kept blowing across my face and I kept pulling it back. In the end I had to hold it, which rather ruined all the photos. Anyway, later I looked at myself and I had pink streaks like whiskers on one side of my face from where the hair had got caught on my lipstick and been dragged across my cheek. The problem was that I'd sat through the entire lunch like this! Then I wiped it all off and had a bare patch on my cheek, and no spare make-up. Don't think I'm silly, but it completely ruined the day for me. I so wanted to look perfect, and I didn't.'

JILLY is 17, and at school
'I had been at the gym, but was meeting friends in the bar upstairs afterwards. I got showered and changed, and put on tights, a floaty long skirt and a jacket. I felt good, and was pleased with how I looked.

'I went to leave the gym, and went past a group of lads on the exercise bikes. I started to go up the stairs and could see in the mirrors that the lads were all looking at me, and I have to admit I loved it. As I walked into the bar, I ran a hand behind my skirt and to my horror it wasn't there! Just my legs! My skirt had got caught in my waistband and my bottom was showing, but the fabric was so flimsy I just hadn't felt it. I quickly pulled it down and nobody noticed, but every time I see those lads now I blush. They weren't admiring me, they were studying my bottom and laughing at me. I double-check everything now.'

And finally, may I add my own personal all-time cringer? I have narrow shoulders and under certain sweaters I some-times wear those shoulder pads which have velcro on the back, so they're not permanent fixtures.

• • • • • • • • • • • •

I was at a casual function wearing trousers, a shirt and a sweater, and as it got hot I removed the sweater. A full two hours later I went to the ladies' loo and saw one of the shoulder pads sitting just on the side of my head, very obvious, as it was a pale yellow and my hair is very dark. It had become detached when I removed the sweater and the velcro had stuck to my hair. What I can never get over even now, or understand, is why nobody pointed it out to me! I had been talking animatedly, and laughing a lot, and it must have been dancing and bobbing about like anything, yet nobody said a word!

• • • • • • • • • • • • •

Recipes

•••••••••••••••

Main Meals

Country Chicken Casserole

Serves 4   Calories per serving: 290

1 tablespoon vegetable oil
2 skinless, boneless chicken breasts
  or legs
1 small onion, finely chopped
2 leeks, cut into rounds
8 small whole carrots

1 tablespoon cornflour
450 ml/15 fl oz chicken stock
100 ml/3½ fl oz skimmed milk
salt and freshly ground black pepper
1 tablespoon wholegrain mustard

1   Preheat the oven to 170°C/325°F/Gas Mark 3.

2   Heat a little of the oil in a large frying-pan, add the chicken pieces and cook over a high heat, turning, for 1 minute. Then transfer to an ovenproof casserole dish.

3   Add the onion to the frying-pan and stir-fry for 1–2 minutes until golden. Add to the chicken with the leeks and carrots.

4   Heat the remaining oil in a small saucepan and stir in the cornflour. Cook over a medium heat for 1 minute, stirring, then gradually add the stock, stirring all the time.

5   Add the milk, salt and pepper.

6   Pour over the chicken and cook in the oven for 45 minutes.

7   Transfer to a serving plate, reserving the sauce. Stir the mustard into the sauce and pour over the chicken.

Chicken Breast with Potatoes Anna

Serves 2   Calories per serving: 497

2 skinless, boneless chicken breasts	25 g/1 oz butter
a few basil leaves, finely chopped	salt and freshly ground black pepper
heaped tablespoon crème fraîche	1 clove garlic, crushed
400 g/14 oz potatoes, peeled and	2 tablespoons olive oil
sliced into rounds	salad or baby asparagus to serve

1   Preheat the oven to 180°C/350°F/Gas Mark 4.

2   Steep the basil leaves in the crème fraîche and set aside in a small bowl.

3   Meanwhile, arrange the thinly-sliced potatoes in layers in an ovenproof dish, dotting each layer with a little butter and sprinkling with salt, pepper and garlic.

4   Place the chicken breasts in a separate ovenproof dish and brush with a little olive oil. Cover each dish with foil and place in the oven.

5   After about 25 minutes, remove the foil from both dishes, pour the crème fraîche and basil mixture over the chicken and brush a little more oil over the top of the potatoes.

6   Turn up the heat to 200°C/400°F/Gas Mark 6 to cook for up to 10 more minutes, checking that your potatoes are not over-browning, nor the chicken liquid boiling.

7   Serve immediately, with a green salad or baby asparagus.

Chicken Roulade with Layered Vegetables

Serves 4   Calories per serving: 260

Don't be put off by the elaborate-sounding name of this dish. Chicken Roulade is terribly simple to make and also looks very impressive. You should really blanch the watercress before using it, but I never do and it still comes out perfectly. The layered vegetables look great and add the necessary moistness.

• • • • • • • • • • • • • •

4 skinless, boneless chicken breasts	400 g/14 oz potatoes, mashed
2–3 bunches watercress (depending on size)	400 g/14 oz broccoli, boiled and mashed
a little butter	400 g/14 oz carrot or carrot and swede, boiled and mashed
salt and freshly ground black pepper	

1   Preheat the oven to 170°C/325°F/Gas Mark 3.

2   Place the chicken breasts on a non-stick board, cover with clingfilm and beat each one with a rolling pin until flattened out to about 15 cm/6 in square.

3   Cut off the watercress stalks and discard. Rinse the leaves and drain thoroughly.

4   Divide the watercress between the chicken breasts. Dot with the butter and season with salt and pepper.

5   Starting at one edge, firmly fold up the chicken breast around the watercess, pressing the cress down and bringing in the sides to form a parcel. Tie firmly with string.

6   When you have parcelled up all 4 chicken breasts, lay them in an ovenproof dish and cover tightly with foil. Cook in the oven for about 40 minutes.

7   Meanwhile, layer the vegetables in a wide, shallow dish. Start with a layer of mashed potato, then broccoli, carrot and potato again, until you have used up all the vegetables. Finish with a top layer of potato.

8   Brush the top with a little melted butter and place in the oven once the chicken has been cooking for 15 minutes.

9   When the chicken is cooked, untie the string and slice each breast into medallions. Place on a serving plate. They should look like attractive pinwheels with a green centre.

10   Serve immediately, with the vegetables, which will be ready at the same time as the chicken.

Chicken Supreme with Basmati Rice

Serves 2   Calories per serving: 403

---

100 g/4 oz Basmati rice	pinch of paprika
1 tablespoon vegetable oil	salt and freshly ground black pepper
1 small onion, finely chopped	1 clove garlic, crushed (optional)
100 g/4 oz mushrooms, sliced	2 tablespoons low-fat crème fraîche
2 skinless, boneless chicken breasts, cut into thin strips	chopped fresh parsley, to garnish

---

1   Cook the rice according to the packet instructions. Drain and reserve.

2   Heat the oil in a frying-pan, add the onion and mushrooms and cook for about 2 minutes, until soft.

3   Sprinkle the chicken strips with paprika, salt and pepper. Add to the pan and stir-fry until cooked through (the chicken should be white in the middle – test by cutting into a strip).

4   Add the garlic, if using.

5   Add the crème fraîche, stir and turn up the heat for 30 seconds. Turn on to a serving plate, spoon the rice around and garnish with the parsley.

Chicken Biryani

Serves 4   Calories per serving: 378

This is a lovely 'dry' chicken curry dish, which is ideally suited to slimmers. It is also ready in no time at all!

---

4 skinless, boneless chicken breasts	1 teaspoon coriander seeds, crushed
2 tablespoons vegetable oil	1 teaspoon garam masala
1 small onion, finely chopped	1 teaspoon dried garlic granules
100 g/4 oz dry weight Basmati rice	(optional)
1 teaspoon ground cumin	

---

1   Cut the chicken into very thin strips. Brush with a little of the oil.

• • • • • • • • • • • • • •

2   Heat the remaining oil in a large frying-pan or wok.

3   Add the onion and fry over a low heat until transparent.

4   Cook the rice according to the packet instructions.

5   Combine the spices in a small bowl.

6   Toss the chicken strips in the spices, making sure they are completely covered and you have used all the spices.

7   Add the chicken to the frying-pan, turning quickly to seal. Keeping the heat low, stir-fry for 3–5 minutes with the onion.

8   When the chicken is white in the middle (test by cutting into a strip), turn up the heat and gently brown the strips on all sides.

9   Drain the rice and return to the pan. Add the chicken mixture to the rice and combine quickly.

10   Serve immediately with a green salad.

Mexican Chilli Chicken

Serves 4   Calories per serving: 315

1½ tablespoons vegetable oil	1 x 400 g/14 oz tin chopped tomatoes
4 skinless, boneless chicken breasts	2 tablespoons wine vinegar
1 clove garlic, finely chopped	1 teaspoon Tabasco sauce
1 onion, finely chopped	1 teaspoon brown sugar
2 fresh chillies, finely chopped	1 avocado, halved, stoned and cut
1 green pepper, chopped	into chunks
a few fresh coriander leaves, chopped	juice of 1 lime
½ teaspoon ground coriander	salt and freshly ground black pepper

1   Heat ½ tablespoon of the oil in a large frying-pan, add the chicken and cook on all sides until browned. Transfer to a shallow ovenproof dish.

2   Preheat the oven to 190°C/375°F/Gas Mark 5.

3   Heat the remaining oil in the frying-pan, add the garlic, onion, chillies and green pepper and cook over a low heat until just soft.

4   Add the coriander, tomatoes, vinegar, Tabasco and sugar. Stir and simmer gently for 20 minutes until thick.
5   Toss the avocado chunks in the lime juice.
6   Pour the sauce over the chicken breasts. Bake in the oven, uncovered, for 25 minutes.
7   Remove from the oven and gently stir in the avocado.
8   Return to the oven and cook for a further 10 minutes.

Spicy Chicken with Chilli-fried Red Rice

Serves 4   Calories per serving: 325

4 skinless, boneless chicken breasts	300 g/10 oz red rice, cooked
	squeeze of lemon juice
For the rice	soy sauce
3 tablespoons vegetable oil	freshly ground black pepper
6 spring onions, peeled and sliced	
2 teaspoons grated fresh root ginger	*For the marinade*
1 teaspoon finely chopped lemon	3 tablespoons soy sauce
grass	2 tablespoons oil
2 cloves garlic, crushed (optional)	juice of 1 lime
1 red chilli pepper, de-seeded and	1 clove garlic, crushed
finely chopped	2 teaspoons 5-spice powder

1   Place the chicken breasts in a dish.
2   Mix the marinade ingredients and pour over the chicken. Leave for 30 minutes.
3   For the rice, heat 2 tablespoons of the oil in a frying-pan and fry the spring onions, ginger, lemon grass, garlic and chilli pepper.
4   Stir in the cooked rice, lemon juice and soy sauce. Season with black pepper, toss well and reserve, keeping hot.
5   Lift the chicken from the marinade. Heat the remaining oil in the frying pan and fry the chicken until browned on both sides. Lower the heat and continue cooking until cooked through. Slice each breast thickly and arrange on plates.

• • • • • • • • • • • • • •

6   Pour the remaining marinade into a pan, bring to the boil and add a dash of soy sauce. Spoon over the chicken and serve with the rice and a mixed green salad or green vegetables.

Cod in Lemon Caper Sauce with Lime Rice

Serves 4   Calories per serving: 304

4 skinless cod fillets	2 tablespoons capers
1 teacup skimmed milk	2 tablespoons chopped fresh parsley
salt and freshly ground white pepper	2 tablespoons fresh double cream
1 tablespoon plain flour	100 g/4 oz long-grain rice
25 g/1 oz butter	grated zest of 1 lime
1 teaspoon grated lemon zest	

1   Place the cod fillets in a large frying-pan, add the milk and season with salt and pepper. Cover with a lid and poach gently for about 10 minutes, until the fish is cooked through. Remove the fish from the milk and set aside, keeping warm.

2   Add the flour to the warm milk, stirring constantly to prevent lumps forming. Add the butter and lemon zest. Keep stirring as the sauce thickens.

3   Stir in the capers, parsley and cream. Season to taste with salt and pepper.

4   Meanwhile, cook the rice according to the packet instructions. Drain. Stir the lime zest into the rice.

5   Spoon the rice on to a serving dish. Top with the cod fillets and pour the sauce over the top. Serve with green vegetables.

Salmon with Mashed Potatoes and Green Vegetables

Serves 1   Calories per serving: 516

1 salmon fillet	1 teaspoon butter
175 g/6 oz potatoes	broccoli, mangetout, French beans or
a little skimmed milk	peas (or a mixture)
salt and freshly ground black pepper	chopped fresh parsley, to garnish
chopped fresh tarragon or pinch dried	
tarragon	

1 Preheat the oven to 190°C/375°F/Gas Mark 5.

2 Place the salmon fillet in a greased, ovenproof dish and cook in the oven for 10–15 minutes.

3 Boil the potatoes. When cooked, remove from pan, drain and mash with the milk. Season to taste with salt and pepper.

4 To make the tarragon butter, mix the tarragon with softened butter.

5 When the fish is nearly ready, put on your chosen vegetables to boil or steam.

6 Serve the salmon fillet immediately with a pat of tarragon butter, garnished with parsley.

Poached Cod or Salmon Parcel

Serves 1   Calories per serving: 300

This recipe is very easy and ideal for working people who want to avoid fast takeaway food. Ready-cut vegetable batons are available from supermarkets. Use any combination of vegetables you like, but try to go for vegetables with a high water content.

2 teaspoons vegetable oil	7 g/¼ oz butter
1 courgette, cut into batons	a few chopped fresh tarragon leaves
1 carrot, cut into batons	or pinch dried tarragon, if using
1 x 100 g/4 oz skinless cod or salmon	salmon
fillet	salt and freshly ground black pepper

• • • • • • • • • • • • •

1   Preheat the oven to 190°C/375°F/Gas Mark 5.

2   Brush a 30 cm/12 in square of greaseproof paper with some of the oil and place on a baking sheet.

3   Place the vegetable batons on the greaseproof, top with the fish, add the butter and pour the remaining oil over. If you are using salmon, add the tarragon.

4   Seal the paper by lifting and folding together the two opposite sides, and tuck underneath.

5   Cook the parcel in the oven for 10–15 minutes. Serve with 3–4 mashed or boiled potatoes.

Seafood Pilaff

Serves 4   Calories per serving: 316

$\frac{1}{2}$ teaspoon ground turmeric	50 g/ 2 oz French beans
$\frac{1}{2}$ teaspoon dried chillies	1 clove garlic, crushed
3 cloves	225 g/8 oz dry weight Basmati rice
3 cardamom pods	100 g/4 oz scallops
300 ml/10 fl oz fish stock	100 g/4 oz prawns
90 ml/3 fl oz white wine	3 tablespoons sour cream or single
1 tablespoon olive oil	cream
1 leek, sliced	2 spring onions, thinly sliced
1 courgette, sliced	

1   Preheat the oven to 190°C/375°F/Gas Mark 5.

2   Combine the spices in a small bowl.

3   Boil the stock and wine together in a pan.

4   Heat the oil in a large frying-pan or wok. Add the vegetables and garlic and leave to sweat for 1 minute, turning.

5   Add the rice and combined spices. Cook for 2–3 minutes, or until translucent.

6   Pour the boiling stock on to the rice and vegetables and simmer for 5 minutes. Stir in the seafood, cover and cook over a very low heat for 20 minutes, checking regularly that the mixture is not burning.

7   The pilaff is ready when all the liquid is absorbed. Let it stand for a minute, then fluff it up with a fork. Mix in the cream and sprinkle with the spring onions.

Crunchy Seafood Gratin

Serves 4   Calories per serving: 365

3 slices stale wholemeal bread, crusts removed
2 teaspoons groundnut oil
2 leeks, sliced
1 clove garlic, peeled and lightly bruised
700 ml/1¼ pints skimmed milk
salt and freshly ground black pepper
200 g/7 oz haddock, cod or coley fillet, skinned
100 g/4 oz small mushrooms, halved

400 g/14 oz frozen mixed seafood, thawed
pinch of seafood seasoning
40 g/1½ oz low-fat spread
40 g/1½ oz plain flour
1 teaspoon lemon juice
1 teaspoon mustard powder
2 tablespoons half-fat cream
2 tablespoons grated half-fat Cheddar-style cheese

1   Shred the bread on a coarse grater or simply chop into small pieces. Heat the oil in a non-stick frying-pan, add the leeks and garlic and, over a very high heat, stir-fry for 1 minute. Remove with a slotted spoon to a plate.
2   Add the bread to the pan and stir for 1 minute. (There will be hardly any oil left in the pan when you do this.) When the bread is just taking on a darker colour, remove from the pan and set aside.
3   Pour the milk into the frying-pan, season with salt and pepper, and add the fish, leeks, garlic and mushrooms. Poach gently for 10 minutes, then add the mixed seafood and cook for a further 1–2 minutes.
4   Strain the milk into a jug, then flake the fish and arrange it, with the seafood, leeks and mushrooms in a large gratin dish, discarding the garlic. Sprinkle the seafood seasoning over and keep warm.
5   Melt the low-fat spread in a saucepan and add the flour. Stir for 1 minute, then gradually add the strained milk, stirring all the time.

• • • • • • • • • • • • •

6   When you have a smooth sauce, stir in the lemon juice, mustard and cream, check the seasoning and pour over the fish and vegetables. Sprinkle the bread, and then the cheese, on top. Put under a medium grill for 4–5 minutes to heat through and brown the topping.

Kedgeree

Serves 2   Calories per serving: about 390

You might think the calorie content of this dish is high, but served as a main meal, with a green salad or other vegetables, it makes a slightly exotic nourishing and tasty meal, and allows you a good 1,000 calories for the rest of the day. Alternatively, served as a light lunch dish, or traditionally as a breakfast dish, you could halve the quantities given. Train yourself to eat less, try having half now and half later – you may find you don't want the second portion.

2 × 225 g/8 oz smoked haddock fillets	1–2 teaspoons mild curry powder
skimmed milk, to poach	1 teaspoon ground turmeric
100 g/4 oz dry weight white Basmati rice	pinch freshly grated nutmeg
	pinch cayenne pepper
7 g/¼ oz butter	2 hard-boiled eggs
½ onion, finely chopped	salt and freshly ground black pepper

1   Place the haddock in an ovenproof dish or large frying-pan. Cover with milk and poach gently until softened through.
2   Meanwhile cook the rice according to the packet instructions. Drain thoroughly.
3   In another frying-pan, melt the butter, add the onion and fry gently until soft. Add the drained rice, curry powder, turmeric, nutmeg and cayenne, and stir.
4   Remove the haddock when cooked, reserving the milk and flake the fish. Add the fish to the rice mixture.
5   Shell the hard-boiled eggs and cut into quarters. Add to the rice and fish mixture.

6   Strain in the milk from the poached fish. Stir everything together, adjust the seasoning and serve hot.

Pasta Primavera

Serves 1   Calories per serving: 278

---

50 g/2 oz fresh pasta spirals or quills
1 tablespoon olive oil
handful mixed mangetout, baby
   sweetcorn, sugar-snap peas, carrot
   sticks, red and green peppers,
   beansprouts

1 teaspoon pesto sauce
2 teaspoons crème fraîche
salt and freshly ground black pepper

---

1   Cook the pasta according to the packet instructions. Drain and keep warm.
2   Heat the oil in a deep frying-pan or wok, and add the mixed vegetables. Toss over a high heat for 1 minute.
3   Add the pasta and the pesto sauce. Turn for 30 seconds.
4   Remove from the heat, add the crème fraîche, season to taste with salt and pepper and serve immediately.

Spaghetti with Smoked Salmon, Dill and Watercress

Serves 2   Calories per serving: 236

---

100 g/4 oz fresh spaghetti
1 teaspoon olive oil or 15 g/½ oz
   butter
2 slices smoked salmon, cut into thin
   strips

salt and freshly ground black pepper
1 tablespoon crème fraîche
1 bunch watercress, washed and
   stripped into sprigs
1 teaspoon dried dill

---

1   Cook the spaghetti according to the packet instructions. Drain.
2   Heat the oil or butter in a large frying-pan. Add the salmon and cook for 30 seconds, stirring constantly.
3   Add the spaghetti to the salmon, season with salt and pepper, and stir in the crème fraîche. Heat through again

and stir in the watercress and dill. Serve immediately on hot plates.

Linguini in Creamy Watercress Sauce

Serves 2   Calories per serving: 361

1 tablespoon vegetable oil	150 ml/5 fl oz single cream
1 medium onion, finely chopped	2 bunches firmly packed watercress,
1 clove garlic, crushed (optional)	trimmed
125 ml/4 fl oz dry white wine	225 g/8 oz linguini
125 ml/4 fl oz fish stock	salt and freshly ground black pepper
1 teaspoon cornflour	

1   Heat the oil in a large pan. Add the onion and garlic and cook over a low heat until soft.

2   Add the wine and stock and boil until reduced by one third, stirring continuously.

3   Blend the cornflour with a little of the cream. Add with the remaining cream to the pan and keep stirring until the mixture thickens.

4   Remove from the heat and add the watercress. You can blend the sauce in a food processor if you prefer it smooth.

5   Meanwhile, cook the linguini according to the packet instructions and add to the sauce in the pan. Season to taste with salt and pepper. Serve immediately.

Macaroni Cheese with Tomatoes

Serves 4   Calories per serving: 488

150 g/5 oz macaroni	23 g/1 oz Parmesan cheese, freshly
25 g/1 oz cornflour	grated
600 ml/1 pint skimmed milk	salt and freshly ground black pepper
25 g/1 oz Edam or Cheddar cheese,	2 large tomatoes sliced
grated	

1   Preheat the oven to 200°C/400°F/Gas Mark 6.

2   Cook the macaroni according to the packet instructions. Drain thoroughly and place in a greased, shallow, wide ovenproof dish.

3   To make the sauce, blend the cornflour with a cup of milk in a saucepan until you have a smooth paste. Heat, stirring continuously, until the mixture thickens. Gradually add the remaining milk. Turn the heat up and bring the sauce to a gentle boil, stirring continuously for 30 seconds to allow the cornflour to cook.

4   Remove from the heat and add the Edam or Cheddar cheese, reserving a little. Stir until melted.

5   Add the Parmesan cheese and season to taste with salt and pepper.

6   Pour the sauce over the macaroni and stir. Top with the tomatoes and the remaining grated cheese. Cook in the oven for about 20 minutes until browned.

Money Bags

Makes 12   Calories per serving of 6: 516

100 g/4 oz ricotta cheese	filo pastry
25 g/ 1 oz Parmesan cheese, freshly grated	melted butter for brushing

1   Preheat the oven to 200°C/400°F/Gas Mark 6.

2   Mix together the ricotta and Parmesan cheese.

3   Cut the filo into 12 cm/5 in squares. Brush one square with melted butter and place another on top at an angle. Spoon the cheese filling on to the middle and gather up the edges, pressing them together to make a pouch. Brush with melted butter, place on a baking sheet and repeat.

4   Bake in the oven for about 5 minutes, until golden and crisp.

Mushroom Medley Risotto

Serves 2   Calories per serving: 323

400 g/14 oz dry weight risotto rice	2 teaspoons tomato purée
15 g/½ oz butter	2 tablespoons half-fat crème fraîche
1 onion, finely chopped	salt and freshly ground black pepper
1 clove garlic, crushed	pinch of nutmeg
400 g/14 oz mushrooms, sliced	pinch of paprika

1   Cook the rice according to the packet instructions.

2   Melt the butter in a large frying-pan. Add the onion and garlic and cook over a low heat until transparent.

3   Add the mushrooms. Keep stirring until coated with the butter.

4   Add the rice and stir in the tomato purée and crème fraîche. Add the salt, pepper and nutmeg and cook for a further 2–3 minutes. Sprinkle with paprika and serve immediately.

Omelette Spanish or Herb

Serves 1   Calories per serving: about 220

2 eggs	red and green pepper, onion,
salt and freshly ground black pepper	mushrooms, cold potato (for the
7 g/¼ oz butter	Spanish omelette)
mixed fresh herbs, chopped (for the herb omelette)	

1   Beat the eggs lightly in a bowl. Season with salt and pepper.

2   Heat the butter in a medium frying-pan until hot but not blackened.

3   *For the herb omelette* Add the eggs, covering the bottom of the pan quickly. Using a fork, draw the edges of the omelette into the centre, letting the liquid run to the outside. Keep this up until the omelette is beginning to set but is still moist. Add the herbs, fold over and serve immediately.

• • • • • • • • • • • • •

4 *For the Spanish omelette* Add the chopped vegetables to the butter and stir together for a minute. Add the eggs and cook on the bottom only. Cook the top of the omelette by holding under a medium grill until set.

Vegetable Chilli

Serves 4   Calories per serving: 280

225 g/8 oz dry weight Basmati rice	2 fresh green chillies, de-seeded and finely chopped
1 tablespoon vegetable oil	1 teaspoon dried chillies (optional)
1 small onion, finely chopped	1 x 200 g/7 oz tin kidney beans, drained
1 large cold potato, cubed	
1 red pepper, de-seeded and chopped	1 x 400 g/14 oz tin chopped tomatoes
1 green pepper, de-seeded and chopped	2 tablespoons tomato purée
handful of cooked, sliced French or runner beans	small dot of butter
	salt and freshly ground black pepper
other vegetables (optional)	chopped fresh parsley, to garnish

1   Cook the rice according to the packet instructions.

2   Heat the oil in a large frying-pan, add the onion and potato and fry gently until slightly browned.

3   Add the peppers, beans and any other vegetables, if using.

4   Stir for about 1 minute, until heated through. Add the fresh chillies, and the dried chillies, if using, the kidney beans, tomatoes and tomato purée.

5   Keeping the heat low, simmer gently for a further 3 minutes, stirring occasionally.

6   Drain the cooked rice, add a small dot of butter and stir through, to keep the rice shiny and the grains separated. Turn on to a serving dish.

7   Season the vegetables with salt and pepper to taste and add to the rice. Garnish with parsley.

• • • • • • • • • • • • • •

Cauliflower Cheese

Serves 2   Calories per serving: 309

Like macaroni cheese, cauliflower cheese is one of the nation's favourites, which slimmers always think they have to do without. This recipe omits the usual butter content of traditional cauliflower cheese, but by using full-flavoured mature cheese, you will sacrifice none of the taste.

1 head cauliflower	75 g/3 oz strong cheese, such as
300 ml/10 fl oz skimmed milk	Cheddar, Leicester, Cheshire,
1 bayleaf	grated
2 teaspoons cornflour	salt and freshly ground black pepper

1   Pour 5 cm/2 in water into a large saucepan. Wash the cauliflower and remove any discoloured or wilted outer leaves

2   Make a cut in the shape of a cross in the base of the cauliflower, to allow the water to penetrate. Place in the pan and cover with a tightly fitting lid. Bring to the boil and allow to simmer.

3   Reserve 2 tablespoons of the milk and put the remainder with the bayleaf into a saucepan. Bring to a slow simmer.

4   Combine the cornflour and the reserved milk in a cup and stir to a smooth paste. As the milk begins to boil, add the cornflour mixture and stir well.

5   Stir continuously as the mixture begins to thicken. Remove from the heat, discard the bayleaf and stir in most of the grated cheese, reserving a handful for the topping. Season the sauce with salt and pepper.

6   To test the cauliflower, cut straight downwards with a sharp, long knife. It should feel soft but firm. Drain and place in an ovenproof dish.

7   Pour the sauce over the cauliflower and sprinkle with the reserved grated cheese. Place under a hot grill for a few minutes until the cheese begins to bubble and turn brown.

8   Serve immediately with boiled or jacket potatoes.

Courgette and Tomato Gratin

Serves 2   Calories per serving: 248

---

25 g/1 oz butter
3 tablespoons olive oil
675 g/1½ lb courgettes, thinly sliced
1 medium onion, chopped
1 clove garlic, chopped

450 g/1 lb fresh tomatoes, peeled and
    roughly chopped
salt and freshly ground black pepper
25 g/1 oz soft fresh breadcrumbs

---

1   Preheat the oven to 200°C/400°F/Gas Mark 6.

2   Melt the butter with 1 tablespoon of the oil in a large saucepan over a medium heat, add the courgettes, cover and cook for 5–7 minutes, until just tender to the point of a knife. You may need to cook the courgettes in two batches, depending on the size of the pan.

3   Meanwhile, heat the remaining oil in a medium-large saucepan over a medium heat, add the onion, cover and cook for 5 minutes. Add the garlic and cook for 1 further minute.

4   Reduce the heat under the onion, add the tomatoes, cover and cook for about 15 minutes, until they have collapsed and any water they give off has evaporated. Season well with salt and pepper.

5   Stir the courgettes into the tomato mixture and pour into a shallow, lightly greased, ovenproof dish. Level the top, sprinkle with breadcrumbs and dot with the remaining butter.

6   Bake, uncovered, in the oven for 25–30 minutes, until the top is golden-brown and crisp. Serve immediately.

Variations

Leek gratin: Replace the courgettes with the same weight of trimmed leeks. Slice the leeks thinly and cook gently in the butter and oil for about 15 minutes, until tender. Add to the tomato mixture and continue as above.

Parsnip, Potato or Kohlrabi Gratin: Replace the courgettes

• • • • • • • • • • • • • •

with the same weight of parsnips, potatoes or kohlrabi, cut into slices about 5 mm/¼ in thick and steam or boil until just tender. Arrange the vegetables in the casserole dish in layers, spreading each layer with the tomato mixture. Proceed as above.

Cashew Nut Korma

Serves 4   Calories per serving: 394

75 g/3 oz creamed coconut, cut into flakes
2 tablespoons sunflower oil
2 medium onions, chopped
2 fresh green chillies, de-seeded and thinly sliced
2 cloves garlic, chopped
½ teaspoon ground cumin
½ teaspoon ground tumeric
½ teaspoon ground coriander
100 g/4 oz cashew nuts, puréed in a blender or finely ground in a mouli

salt and freshly ground black pepper
225 g/8 oz long-grain white or brown rice
½ medium cauliflower, divided into florets
100 g/4 oz courgettes, sliced
100 g/4 oz frozen peas
2–4 tablespoons chopped fresh coriander

1 Put the coconut into a bowl and cover with 450 ml/15 fl oz boiling water. Stir, then leave to dissolve completely.

2 Meanwhile, heat the oil in a large saucepan over a medium heat, add the onions, cover and cook for 5–7 minutes until tender.

3 Add the chillies, garlic and spices, stir well and cook for a further 1–2 minutes. Remove from the heat and set aside.

4 Stir the cashew nuts into the bowl containing the coconut. Add this mixture to the onion mixture and season with salt and pepper. Cover and set aside once more.

5 Cook the rice. When it is almost ready, cook the vegetables. Pour 1 cm/½ in boiling water into a large saucepan, add the cauliflower, cover and half-boil, half-steam for 1 minute. Add the courgettes, cover again and cook for 3 minutes. Drain.

6   Stir the vegetables into the creamy cashew nut mixture along with the peas. Warm through over a low heat. Check the seasoning and serve, sprinkled with coriander, with the rice.

NOTE: *You can prepare ahead to the end of stage 4. The coconut and cashew mixture will keep for up to 24 hours in a covered container in the refrigerator.*

Thai-Style Stir-Fried Vegetables

Serves 4   Calories per serving: 221

2 tablespoons oil	1 fresh green chilli, de-seeded and
225 g/8 oz beansprouts	finely chopped
100 g/4 oz baby sweetcorn	1–2 whole pods of star anise, seeds
100 g/4 oz mangetout, trimmed	removed and crushed
small bunch of spring onions,	1 tablespoon soy sauce
chopped	finely grated zest and juice of 1 lime
1 red pepper, cored, de-seeded and	2–3 tablespoons chopped fresh
thinly sliced	coriander
100 g/4 oz button mushrooms, sliced,	100 g/4 oz dry weight Thai Jasmine
or straw mushrooms from a jar or	or Basmati rice
can, kept whole	
1 stalk of lemon grass, white part,	
thinly sliced	

1   Pour the oil into a wok or a large frying-pan and place over a high heat.

2   When the oil is smoking hot, drop in all the vegetables, the lemon grass, chilli and star anise seeds. As the vegetables fry, stir them vigorously with a long-handled wooden spoon until they are evenly heated through but still crisp, about 2 minutes.

3   Add the soy sauce, lime zest and juice and coriander all at once. Stir again over the heat while they sizzle, just a few seconds.

• • • • • • • • • • • • • •

4   Serve with Jasmine or Basmati rice, cooked according to the packet instructions.

Spiced Vegetable Triangles

Makes 8   Calories per serving of 4: 440

1 tablespoon olive oil
1 medium onion, finely chopped
½ teaspoon grated fresh ginger
½ teaspoon cumin seeds
½ teaspoon ground coriander
100 g/4 oz potato, finely diced
100 g/4 oz carrot, finely diced

100 g/4 oz frozen peas
2 tablespoons chopped fresh
   coriander
salt and freshly ground black pepper
4 sheets filo pastry
melted butter for brushing

1   Heat the oil in a large saucepan over a medium heat, add the onion, cover and cook for 5 minutes until tender. Add the spices, potato and carrot, cover and cook for 5–10 minutes, until the vegetables are tender. Stir occasionally, and add a tablespoon or so of water if the mixture sticks.
2   Add the peas and stir until they are thawed. Add the fresh coriander, salt and pepper.
3   Preheat the oven to 200°C/400°F/Gas Mark 6.
4   Cut a sheet of filo pastry lengthways into 2 strips. Spoon filling on to the top edge of one strip and make a triangle, folding the pastry over the filling and then turning this triangle down the length of the filo strip. Brush with melted butter, place on a baking sheet and repeat.
5   Bake the triangles in the oven for about 15 minutes, until golden and crisp.

Light Meals

Herby Stuffed Tomatoes

Serves 4   Calories per serving: 176

---

1 shallot or small onion, finely
  chopped
3 tablespoons chopped fresh flat-leaf
  parsley
1 teaspoon chopped fresh thyme

50 g/2 oz dried breadcrumbs
2 tablespoons olive oil
4 beefsteak tomatoes
salt and freshly ground black pepper

---

1   Preheat the oven to 180°C/350°F/Gas Mark 4. (Alternatively, use a hot grill.)

2   In a bowl, mix together the onion, parsley, thyme, breadcrumbs and oil. (If you have a food processor, put the unchopped onion, parsley and thyme into it along with the breadcrumbs and olive oil and chop finely to combine.)

3   Slice the tops off the tomatoes and reserve them. Scoop out the seeds with a small teaspoon to make a cavity for stuffing. You will not need the inner flesh of the tomatoes for this recipe but you can chop it and add it to a salad, soup or sauce.

4   Season the inside of the tomatoes with salt and pepper. Spoon in the stuffing, stand the tomatoes in a greased ovenproof dish and replace the tops. Cook in the oven or under a hot grill for about 15 minutes, or until the tomatoes are thoroughly heated through but not collapsing. Serve warm or cold.

Jacket Potato with Coronation Chicken

Serves 1   Calories per serving: 232; with 175 g/6 oz jacket potato: 382

---

1 small skinless, boneless chicken breast (about 75g/3 oz), roasted and cooled
1 teaspoon apricot jam

$\frac{1}{2}$ teaspoon mayonnaise
1–2 teaspoons curry powder
flaked almonds (optional)
1 × 175 g/6 oz baked potato

---

1   Cut the chicken into strips and place in a mixing bowl.
2   Mix together the jam, mayonnaise and curry powder. Add the chicken and combine thoroughly. Add more curry powder if you like it spicy.
3   Mix in the almonds, if using, and serve with a jacket potato and colourful mixed salad.

Salmon and Corn Chowder

Serves 4   Calories per serving: 282

---

15 g/$\frac{1}{2}$ oz butter
1 medium carrot, diced
1 small onion, diced
1 leek, chopped into rounds
225 g/8 oz potatoes, peeled and cubed
600 ml/1 pint skimmed milk
300 ml/10 fl oz water

salt and freshly ground black pepper
1 × 200 g/7 oz tin sweetcorn, drained
1 x 175 g/6 oz salmon fillet, skinned and cubed
150 ml/5 fl oz single cream
handful of chopped fresh parsley

---

1   Melt the butter in a saucepan. Add the carrot, onion and leek and stir until transparent. Add the potato and cook for 1 further minute.
2   Pour in the milk and water. Season well with salt and pepper and simmer for 10 minutes.
3   Add the sweetcorn and the salmon and simmer for a further 3–4 minutes.
4   Stir in the cream and parsley and serve immediately.

• • • • • • • • • • • • •

Welsh Rarebit with Tomatoes

Serves 1   Calories per serving: 198

---

1 large slice bread

45 g/1½ oz Edam or Cheddar cheese,
   grated

1–2 tomatoes, sliced

---

1   Toast the bread on one side.

2   Place the cheese on the bread and top with the tomatoes. Grill until brown. Serve with a mixed salad.

Salads

Warm Spicy Chicken Salad

Serves 3   Calories per serving: 328

---

2 boneless, skinless chicken breasts
pinch of paprika
1 teaspoon dried chillies
1 teaspoon dried garlic granules
1 teaspoon freshly ground black
    pepper

2 tablespoons vegetable oil
salad vegetables, such as lettuce,
    cucumber, grated courgette, carrot
    batons, sliced chicory
1 tablespoon soy sauce

---

1   Cut the chicken breasts into thin strips.

2   Mix the spices in a bowl. Toss the chicken strips in the spice mixture until well coated.

3   Heat the oil in a frying-pan, add the chicken and stir-fry over a medium heat for about 5 minutes, turning constantly.

4   Arrange the salad vegetables on a plate.

5   When the chicken is cooked through (check by cutting into a strip – it should be white, not pink), turn up the heat and fry until slightly scorched – about another 30 seconds.

6   Add the soy sauce and toss. Turn out on to the salad and serve immediately.

Smoked Salmon and Avocado Salad

Serves 2   Calories per serving: 290

---

green salad leaves, such as rocket, lamb's lettuce, frisée, endive
1 medium ripe avocado

2 slices smoked salmon, cut ino fine strips
2 tablespoons vinaigrette dressing

---

1   Arrange a bed of salad leaves on 2 plates.

2   Cut the avocado in half and remove the stone. Peel off the skin and place a half on each plate. Slice the avocado longways and arrange round the plate.

3   Arrange the smoked salmon strips over the avocado. Drizzle with dressing and serve immediately.

Bacon and Walnut Salad

Serves 4   Calories per serving: 204

---

selection of mixed salad leaves
sprigs of fresh flat-leaf parsley (optional)
3 tablespoons walnut oil
1 tablespoon balsamic vinegar

1 clove garlic, skinned and crushed
salt and freshly ground black pepper
100 g/4 oz lean, rindless bacon rashers, diced
50 g/2 oz walnut pieces

---

1   Shred any large salad leaves into small pieces and mix with the parsley, if using, in a salad bowl.

2   Put the oil, vinegar, garlic, salt and pepper into a small bowl.

3   Fry the bacon in its own fat until golden-brown. Drain well, then sprinkle over the salad. Add the walnuts.

4   Whisk the dressing ingredients together until well blended, then pour over the salad. Toss together and serve immediately.

Salade Niçoise

Serves 4   Calories per serving: 344

1 x 200g/7 oz tin tuna in oil, drained
   and flaked
100 g/4 oz fine French beans
100 g/4 oz baby broad beans
6 anchovy fillets
½ cucumber
4 tomatoes
20 black olives
3 hard-boiled eggs, shelled
chicory leaves, to serve

For the dressing
6 tablespoons olive oil
2 tablespoons white wine vinegar
1 clove garlic, peeled and crushed
1 teaspoon Dijon mustard
3 tablespoons chopped fresh flat-leaf
   parsley
salt and freshly ground black pepper

1   Place the dressing ingredients in a screw-topped jar and shake well to combine. Set aside.

2   Place the tuna in a mixing bowl. Halve the French beans and blanch them in boiling, salted water with the broad beans for 3 minutes until just tender. Drain and refresh under cold running water.

3   Cut the anchovy fillets into small pieces and slice the cucumber into batons. Cut the tomatoes into wedges. Add the beans, anchovies, cucumber and tomatoes to the tuna along with the olives. Pour over the dressing and toss gently.

4   Wash and dry the chicory and line a serving dish with the leaves. Spoon the prepared salad into the centre. Cut the eggs into quarters and add to the salad. Serve immediately.

Pasta Salad with Avocado Dressing

Serves 4   Calories per serving: 205

100 g/4 oz pasta shapes
salt and freshly ground black pepper
50 g/2 oz asparagus, trimmed, tips
   removed and stalks cut into 2.5
   cm/1 in pieces
1 courgette, trimmed and sliced

1 large ripe avocado
100 g/4 oz very low-fat fromage frais
½ tablespoon lemon juice
½ clove garlic, peeled and crushed
½ eating apple
1 tablespoon chopped fresh coriander

1   Cook the pasta shapes, according to the packet instructions, adding the asparagus stalk pieces 7 minutes before the end of the cooking time and the courgettes and asparagus tips 2–3 minutes before the end of the cooking time.

2   When the pasta and vegetables are cooked, drain well, and rinse under cold running water, then drain well again. Place in a large bowl.

3   Cut the avocado in half and remove the stone, then scoop out the flesh from one half and mash in a bowl. Add the fromage frais, lemon juice, garlic, salt and pepper and mix well together.

4   Chop the remaining avocado half into small pieces. Core and chop the apple. Pour the avocado dressing over the pasta and add the chopped avocado and apple. Toss together until mixed, then sprinkle with the coriander. Serve immediately.

Salmon and Pasta Salad

Serves 4   Calories per serving: 289

---

175 g/6 oz pasta shapes
225 g/8 oz asparagus
2 tablespoons chopped fresh chervil
    or parsley
grated zest and juice of ½ lemon

4 tablespoons French dressing
175 g/6 oz cooked salmon, flaked
1 tablespoon freshly grated Parmesan
    cheese

---

1   Cook the pasta according to the packet instructions. Drain and rinse under cold running water.

2   Trim the asparagus. Remove the tips and set aside. Cut the stalks into 4 cm/1½ in pieces.

3   Bring a pan of salted water to the boil. Add the asparagus stalks and cook for 3 minutes. Remove. Add the tips to the pan and cook for 2 minutes. Drain and set aside.

4   Add the herbs and lemon zest and juice to the French dressing.

• • • • • • • • • • • • • • •

5   Add the dressing to the pasta. Add the asparagus stalks and salmon and toss gently. Transfer to a serving dish.

6   Arrange the asparagus tips on the top and sprinkle with the Parmesan cheese.

Smoked Chicken and Pesto Pasta Salad

Serves 2   Calories per serving: 345

100 g/4 oz pasta shapes	*For the Pesto dressing*
175 g/6 oz cooked, smoked chicken breast	4 tablespoons pesto sauce
	6 tablespoons vegetable oil
12 cherry tomatoes	2 tablespoons red wine vinegar
4 tablespoons pine nuts, toasted	freshly ground black pepper
175 g/6 oz mixed salad leaves	
sprigs of fresh basil, to garnish	

1   Place all the dressing ingredients in a bowl and whisk to combine.

2   Cook the pasta according to the packet instructions until *al dente*. Drain the pasta and immediately toss it with the prepared dressing. Set aside.

3   Slice the chicken into thin strips and halve the cherry tomatoes. Add to the bowl of pasta along with the pine nuts. Toss well.

4   Wash the lettuce leaves and tear any large leaves in half.

5   Line a serving bowl with the lettuce and spoon the pasta into the centre. Garnish with sprigs of basil and serve immediately.

Wild Rice and Thyme Salad

Serves 4   Calories per serving: 170

75 g/3 oz French beans, trimmed and
    halved
75 g/3 oz broad beans, podded
salt and freshly ground black pepper
25 g/1 oz wild rice
75 g/3 oz long-grain brown rice
1 tablespoon grapeseed oil
25 g/1 oz small button mushrooms,
    wiped

1 tablespoon chopped fresh thyme
$\frac{1}{2}$ tablespoon walnut oil
1 tablespoon white wine vinegar
$\frac{1}{2}$ tablespoon Dijon mustard
salt and freshly ground black pepper
sprigs of fresh thyme, to garnish

1 Cook the French beans in a saucepan of boiling salted water for 10–12 minutes, until just tender. Drain under cold running water and set aside to cool.

2 Cook the broad beans in a saucepan of boiling salted water for 5–7 minutes, until just tender. Drain under cold running water, slipping off the outer skins if wished, and set aside to cool.

3 Place the wild rice in a large saucepan of boiling salted water. Boil for 10 minutes before adding the brown rice. Boil together for a further 25–30 minutes, or until both are just tender. Drain the rice under cold running water.

4 Stir together the French beans, broad beans and rice in a large bowl.

5 Heat the grapeseed oil in a small frying-pan and fry the mushrooms with the thyme for 2–3 minutes. Remove from the heat and stir in the walnut oil, vinegar, mustard, salt and pepper. Add to the rice mixture and stir well. Adjust the seasoning. Cool, cover and refrigerate until required. Serve garnished with sprigs of thyme.

• • • • • • • • • • • • • •

Rice and Kidney Bean Salad

Serves 4   Calories per serving: 270

---

225 g/8 oz long-grain brown rice
salt and freshly ground black pepper
low-fat French dressing, to moisten
1 x 225 g/8 oz tin red kidney beans,
    drained
a few spring onions, trimmed and
    chopped

½ cucumber, diced
2–3 celery sticks, trimmed and sliced
chopped fresh parsley, to garnish
salt and freshly ground black pepper

---

1   Cook the rice according to the packet instructions. Drain.

2   While the rice is still warm, add enough French dressing to moisten and stir in the kidney beans. Leave to cool.

3   Mix in the spring onions, cucumber, celery, parsley, salt and pepper.

Oriental Tofu and Bean Salad

Serves 4   Calories per serving: 214

---

2 tablespoons dark soy sauce
2 tablespoons dry sherry
2 tablespoons orange juice
2.5 cm/1 in piece of fresh root ginger,
    peeled and finely grated
freshly ground black pepper
175 g/6 oz smoked firm tofu
1 tablespoon sesame or vegetable
    oil

1 clove garlic, peeled and finely
    chopped
100 g/4 oz mangetout, trimmed
4 spring onions, finely sliced
½ head Chinese leaves, finely
    shredded
425 g/15 oz tin black-eye beans,
    drained and rinsed

---

1   Put the soy sauce, sherry, orange juice, ginger and pepper into a bowl and mix together. Cut the tofu into 1 cm/½ in cubes and stir it into the mixture. Leave to marinate for 1 hour. Drain the tofu, reserving the marinade.

2   Heat the oil in a large non-stick frying-pan. Add the tofu and cook, stirring, for 2 minutes. Add the garlic, mangetout and spring onions and stir-fry for a further 2 minutes. Transfer to a bowl and leave to cool.

3   Wash and dry the Chinese leaves and put into a large salad bowl.

4   Add the beans and reserved marinade to the cold tofu mixture, mix together and pile on top of the Chinese leaves. Carefully toss the salad before serving.

Spicy Vegetable Salad

Serves 4   Calories per serving: 148

---

100 g/4 oz fromage frais
3 tablespoons low-fat French dressing
¼ teaspoon garam masala
225 g/8 oz new potatoes
175 g/6 oz French beans, trimmed
1 large cauliflower, cut into florets

175 g/6 oz mangetout, trimmed
1 large red pepper, de-seeded and
    quartered
chopped fresh parsley and coriander
lettuce leaves, to serve

---

1   To make the dressing, blend the fromage frais, French dressing and garam masala together in a bowl. Leave to stand.

2   Steam the potatoes for about 25 minutes, the French beans for about 15 minutes, the cauliflower for about 10 minutes and the mangetout for about 5 minutes, until they are all just tender or *al dente*.

3   Grill the pepper, skin side up, under a hot grill until blackened. Cover with a damp tea-towel and leave until cool enough to handle. Peel, discard the skin and slice.

4   Halve the potatoes. Slice the cauliflower florets. Slice the mangetout into diagonal strips. Cut the French beans in half crossways. Combine with the red pepper, parsley and coriander.

5   Mix the vegetables with the dressing. Pile on to a platter lined with the lettuce leaves.

• • • • • • • • • • • • •

Spinach and Avocado in Yogurt Dressing

Serves 4   Calories per serving: 196

225 g/8 oz fresh baby spinach, cleaned and trimmed weight, finely shredded	1 ripe avocado
	4 tablespoons low-fat natural yogurt
	grated lemon zest
50g/2 oz radicchio cleaned, trimmed and finely shredded	1 teaspoon lemon juice
	snipped fresh chives, to garnish
400 g/14 oz tin flageolet beans, drained	salt and freshly ground black pepper

1   Put the spinach into a bowl, together with the radicchio and beans.

2   Cut the avocado in half and remove the stone. Peel and slice the avocado and add to the vegetables.

3   To make the dressing, mix the yogurt with the lemon zest and juice, then add the chives, salt and pepper.

4   Just before serving, stir the dressing through the spinach and avocado until well mixed.

Bombay Potato Salad

Serves 2   Calories per serving: 133

450 g/1 lb small new potatoes, scrubbed	pinch ground cumin
salt and freshly ground black pepper	1 green chilli pepper, de-seeded and chopped (optional)
75 ml/3 fl oz Greek yogurt	sprigs of fresh flat-leaf parsley, to garnish
pinch ground coriander	

1   Cook the potatoes in boiling, salted water for 15–20 minutes until tender.

2   To make the dressing, whisk together the yogurt, spices, salt and pepper.

3   Drain the potatoes and immediately stir into the dressing. Leave to cool, then cover and refrigerate until 20 minutes before required.

4   Just before serving, stir in the chilli, if using. Serve garnished with parsley.

• • • • • • • • • • • • •

Cauliflower, Broccoli and Pepper Salad

Serves 4   Calories per serving: 137

---

100 g/4 oz broccoli, trimmed and cut into florets
100 g/4 oz cauliflower, cut into florets
½ small yellow pepper, de-seeded and thinly sliced
½ small red pepper, de-seeded and thinly sliced

½ clove garlic, peeled and crushed
2 tablespoons water
3 tablespoons lemon juice
salt and freshly ground black pepper
sesame seeds, to garnish

---

1   Blanch the broccoli and cauliflower in a saucepan of boiling water for 3 minutes, then drain and leave to cool. Place the broccoli, cauliflower and peppers in a salad bowl.
2   To make the dressing, whisk the garlic, water, lemon juice, salt and pepper together.
3   Pour the dressing over the salad and toss gently to coat. Cover and refrigerate. Sprinkle with sesame seeds just before serving.

Cucumber and Watercress Salad

Serves 2   Calories per serving: 72

---

1 tablespoon white wine vinegar
½ teaspoon caster sugar
½ tablespoon olive oil
juice of 2 lemons (2 tablespoons)
salt and freshly ground black pepper
½ cucumber, cut into matchstick-sized pieces

½ small bunch spring onions, trimmed and sliced
½ bunch watercress
15 g/½ oz walnuts, chopped

---

1   To make the dressing, whisk together the vinegar, sugar, oil and lemon juice. Season to taste with salt and pepper. Toss the cucumber and spring onions together in the dressing. Cover and refrigerate until required.
2   Divide the watercress into sprigs. Rinse and drain, then refrigerate in a polythene bag.

• • • • • • • • • • • • • • • •

3   Just before serving, toss the cucumber and the spring onions again. Sprinkle the walnuts over and surround with watercress sprigs.

Fresh Spinach and Baby Corn Salad
Serves 4   Calories per serving: 82

175 g/6 oz baby spinach	½ teaspoon caster sugar
75 g/3 oz fresh baby sweetcorn	salt and freshly ground pepper
2 tablespoons olive oil	50 g/2 oz alfalfa sprouts
½ clove garlic, skinned and crushed	½ head of chicory, trimmed and
½ tablespoon white wine vinegar	shredded
1 teaspoon Dijon mustard	

1   Wash the spinach well in several changes of cold water. Remove any coarse stalks. Drain well and pat dry on absorbent kitchen paper.
2   Halve the sweetcorn cobs lengthways. Cook in boiling water for about 3–5 minutes until just tender. Drain under cold running water.
3   To make the dressing, whisk together the oil, garlic, vinegar, mustard and sugar. Season to taste with salt and pepper.
4   Mix together the spinach, sweetcorn, alfalfa sprouts and chicory. Toss in the dressing and serve immediately.

French Frisée Salad with Garlic Croûtons
Serves 4   Calories per serving: 259

175 g/6 oz frisée lettuce	*For the Roquefort dressing*
	3 tablespoons corn oil
For the garlic croûtons	3 tablespoons mayonnaise
4 garlic cloves peeled and crushed	2 tablespoons white wine vinegar
6 tablespoons extra virgin olive oil	2 tablespoons water
salt and freshly ground black pepper	½ teaspoon Dijon mustard
75 g/3 oz white bread, crusts	few drops Worcestershire sauce
removed	salt and freshly ground black pepper
	100 g/4 oz Roquefort cheese

1   Prepare the croûtons. Preheat the oven to 180°C/350°F Gas Mark 4.

2   Place the garlic, oil, salt and pepper in a large bowl and mix well. Cut the bread into 1 cm/½ in cubes and add to the bowl. Toss well to coat.

3   Transfer the bread cubes to a baking sheet and bake on the top shelf of the oven for about 15 minutes until golden. Remove and set aside.

4   Place all the dressing ingredients, except the cheese, in a bowl and whisk to combine. Mash the cheese with a fork and add it, a little at a time, to the dressing, whisking well between each addition.

5   Wash and dry the frisée lettuce and tear into bite-sized pieces. Place in a bowl with half the croûtons, pour over the dressing and toss until evenly coated with dressing.

6   Serve the salad immediately with the remaining croûtons scattered over the top.

Iceberg Lettuce With Creamy Lime Dressing

Serves 4   Calories per serving: 54

½ iceberg lettuce, shredded	grated zest and juice of 1 lime
½ cucumber, finely diced	salt and freshly ground black pepper
4 tablespoons low-calorie mayonnaise	
2 tablespoons very low-fat fromage frais	

1   Wash and dry the lettuce and place in a salad bowl. Add the cucumber.

2   Put the mayonnaise, fromage frais, lime zest and juice, salt and pepper into a bowl. Mix well together.

3   Spoon the dressing over the salad and toss lightly just before serving.

• • • • • • • • • • • • •

Strawberry and Cucumber Salad

Serves 4   Calories per serving: 38

---

1 small cucumber
freshly ground black pepper
200 ml/7 fl oz unsweetened apple
  juice

225g/8 oz strawberries, hulled
sprigs of fresh mint, to garnish

---

1   With the prongs of a fork, scrape down the sides of the cucumber to make a ridged effect. Slice the cucumber very thinly and lay in a shallow dish. Sprinkle with pepper to taste. Pour 150 ml/5 fl oz of the apple juice over and refrigerate for 15 minutes.

2   Slice the strawberries if large; otherwise, cut them in half. Put into a small bowl and pour the remaining apple juice over. Refrigerate for 15 minutes.

3   Drain the cucumber and strawberries and arrange them attractively on a serving dish. Garnish with mint sprigs.

Waldorf Salad

Serves 2   Calories per serving: about 200

---

1 red apple, sliced
2 celery sticks, cut into small strips
20 grapes

12 walnuts
2 tablespoons mayonnaise
lettuce

---

1   Place all the ingredients except the lettuce in a bowl and mix well.

2   Turn out on to a bed of lettuce and serve.

Desserts

Baked Apple and Custard

Serves 1   Calories per serving: 130

---

1 large baking apple   2 tablespoons low-fat custard
handful raisins or sultanas or 1
   teaspoon mincemeat

---

1   Preheat the oven to 200°C/400°F/Gas Mark 6.
2   Remove the core from the apple, leaving the base.
3   Fill the centre with the dried fruit or mincemeat.
4   Place in a small dish and cover tightly with foil.
5   Bake in the oven for 20 minutes, or until soft, depending on the size of the apple.
6   Serve hot with custard.

Baked Banana Suzette

Serves 2   Calories per serving: 140; with fromage frais: 199

---

2 bananas halved lengthways   1 measure Cointreau or Grand
juice of 2 oranges   Marnier (optional)
                                        2 tablespoons low-fat fromage frais

---

1   Preheat the oven to 200°C/400°F/Gas Mark 6
2   Lay the bananas in a shallow ovenproof dish. Pour over the orange juice and liqueur.

3   Cover the dish tightly with foil. Bake in the centre of the oven for 10–15 minutes
4   Serve with the fromage frais.

Poached Pear

Serves 1   Calories per serving: 140

---

1 large pear   a few cloves
1 glass red wine

---

1   Preheat the oven to 190°C/375°F/Gas Mark 5.
2   Keeping the stalk intact, peel the pear and cut it flat across the base to enable it to stand upright in the dish.
3   Pour the wine into an ovenproof dish, place the pear upright in it and sprinkle the cloves into the wine.
4   Cover with foil and cook in the oven for 30 minutes.
5   Alternatively, place the pear and cloves in a deep saucepan and simmer gently for about 10 minutes, or until soft. Remove from the pan, discard the cloves and pour the wine over the pear.
6   Serve chilled with low-fat fromage frais, if liked.

Poached Stuffed Peach

Serves 1   Calories per serving: 108

---

1 ripe peach   juice of 1 orange
small piece of marzipan   ½ glass sweet or dry sherry (optional)

---

1   Preheat the oven to 190°C/375°F/Gas Mark 5.
2   Cut the peach in half and remove the stone.
3   Fill the centre with marzipan and press the two halves of the peach together.
4   Place the peach in a small ovenproof dish and pour over the orange juice, with the sherry if using.
5   Cover the dish with foil. Cook in the oven for about 30 minutes. Serve hot, with crème fraîche if liked.

Rice Pudding

Serves 4   Calories per serving: 147

Rice pudding is equally delicious hot or cold. The calorie content is not at all high, and made with skimmed milk it's full of calcium, protein and starch.

600 ml/1 pint skimmed milk   1½ tablespoon sugar
50 g/2 oz pudding rice

1   Preheat the oven to 180°C/350°F/Gas Mark 4.
2   Put all the ingredients into a saucepan and bring to the boil, stirring.
3   When the mixture is boiling, turn down the heat and simmer for a few minutes, stirring to prevent the mixture becoming a sticky mass.
4   Pour into a lightly greased pudding basin and bake in the oven for 45 minutes.
5   Either serve immediately, with a teaspoon of jam, or cool completely, pour into empty yogurt pots and refrigerate until needed. The pudding can then be microwaved if necessary.

Winter Fruit Salad

Serves 8   Calories per serving: 169

1 x 400 g/14 oz tin prunes in fruit juice   1 x 400 g/14 oz tin pear halves in fruit juice
1 x 400 g/14 oz tin apricots in fruit juice   1 x 400 g/14 oz tin blackberries in fruit juice

1   Combine the contents of the tins of fruit in a bowl, using only the fruit juice from the prunes.
2   You can refrigerate what you do not use for another meal. Each serving should be about 225 g/8 oz in weight. Serve with low-fat fromage frais, if liked.

What About the Future?

Anyone who spends a fortnight eating salads, vegetables, fruit, fish and starch and drinking plenty of water, not to mention exercising every day and attending to her grooming, can hardly fail to look much, much better than she did when she started. The question is, can you keep it up?

There's a difference between keeping up a sensible regime of grooming and diet so you look and feel your best at all times, and being taken over by it. In all the years I have been associated with the fitness world, I've known thousands of people – men as well as women – who have crossed over from normal self-interest and gentle vanity to finding themselves in the grip of an obsession. What is also quite extraordinary is that in the midst of all the dedication to looking good and leading a healthy life, I have never known any of them to appear happy. On the one hand you are impressed and inspired by the dedication to a perfect body, and on the other hand you wonder at the mentality of someone who is terrified of eating something which doesn't comply with their diet. I mean, just who's meant to be in control here?

We all know at least one Miss Perfect who lives an exemplary life. Shunning alcohol, cakes and late nights, her skin is cleansed three times a day and she conditions her hair before tying it back to preserve its perfection so it never actually has any kind of style. Her social life is slotted round her exercise sessions, and while she's generally quiet and intense, she can always be counted on to chip in when she hears anyone talk about food. She knows more than anyone else about nutrition, and has sleepless nights about it.

Invitations she can't avoid are planned well in advance so she can adjust her diet beforehand, though it won't matter that it's Christmas Day and Auntie Mary spent the last week filling those six dozen mince pies. Miss Perfect has no thoughts beyond her own needs, and they certainly don't extend to making an old lady feel needed and appreciated by enjoying her mince pies.

What a waste. The obsessive woman of the 1980s is completely outdated. It doesn't get you a better job, it doesn't endear you to your children, colleagues, neighbours or the opposite sex, and it doesn't make you more friends. To make improving yourself worthwhile, you have to know what to do with it. 'I'm doing it for myself' is just about the most empty phrase the last decade has come up with.

Do it for yourself, yes, but do it to enrich your life, not dominate it. Learn what feeling good feels like, learn the techniques of achieving it *and then let it look after itself.*

Your diet in the future

Eat well in the future, but also eat sensiby and realistically. Have a cake, have some chocolate if that's what you want. Have a glass or two of wine, and don't feel bad about it. The best thing about having got yourself into shape and into a proper eating regime is that your weight *won't fluctuate* in future if you stick with your principles. They are *regularity* and *control.*

What if I go on a weekend binge?

The first thing to do is keep calm. Your body won't put on weight straight away, so go back to Day One of the diet plan and follow it for five to seven days. Keep off the alcohol, biscuits and sweets for that period of time, but keep up your four or five little meals a day, plus lots of water.

• • • • • • • • • • • • • •

Above all, don't panic and miss meals to compensate. It won't work.

If I'm going out to a restaurant for a meal, shouldn't I miss lunch that day to 'make room'?

Definitely not! You see, it's psychological. By missing a couple of meals and going out having eaten little more than a couple of crispbreads, you'll think you can afford to eat as much as you like. Maybe you can, but we now come to the difference between genuine food appreciation and sheer gluttony. Quite simply, you have no need to eat like a horse, and it ruins the image you've been working for. Eat your normal meals, then go out and eat what you truly fancy, not what you've been saving a corner of your stomach for!

How can I look good for ever?

Nobody looks good all the time, and allowing your apperance to take you over is taking it all a bit far. Good grooming is nothing more than common sense; it's also enjoyable to feel happy about your appearance and as you get older you'll have far more compliments. After all, if a twenty-four-year-old looks good it's hardly worthy of comment. When a fifty-year-old looks good it's remarked on and the compliments flow. A lady I know who looks fantastic at sixty-two said to me recently, 'When I was thirty and looked after my skin nobody ever commented. Now I'm a pensioner, suddenly everyone's raving about my complexion. I knew all that hard work would be worth it one day!'

You'll always look good if you remember the golden rules:

1 Stand up straight, chest out, head up.
2 Smile.
3 Keep slim.
4 Eat well.
5 Exercise!

A last word

Whatever you wear, however beautiful your jewellery, your immaculately manicured nails and elaborate hairdo, try always to smile and look as if you're happy and enjoying yourself.

If something goes wrong, if you get a drink spilled over you or the baby is sick on your shoulder or your host's dog jumps up and ladders your tights, laugh it off. You might feel murderous, but people will warm to you and sympathize with you if you appear happy-go-lucky and handle a disaster with style.

Have a good time!

Index of Recipes

• • • • • • • • • • • • •